Health and Social Care Knowledge and Skills

Essential Study Skills for Health and Social Care

Health and Social Care Knowledge and Skills

Essential Study Skills for Health and Social Care

Edited by Marjorie Lloyd and Peggy Murphy

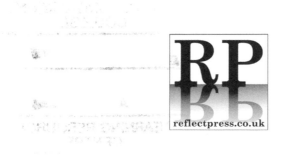

reflectpress.co.uk

First published in 2008

ISBN: 978 1 906052 14 0

British Library Cataloguing in Publication Data
A catalogue record for this book is available from the British Library

Production project management by Deer Park Productions
Typeset by Kestrel Data, Exeter, Devon
Cover design by Oxmed
Printed and bound by Bell & Bain Ltd, Glasgow
Distributed by BEBC, Albion Close, Parkstone, Poole, Dorset BH12 3LL

Published by Reflect Press Ltd
11 Attwyll Avenue
Exeter
Devon, EX2 5HN
UK
01392 204400

www.reflectpress.co.uk

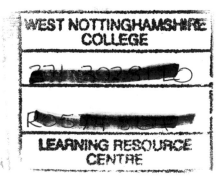

Contents

Health and Social Care Series

Series Editors: Sue Cuthbert, Jan Quallington and Elaine Donnelly – all at the University of Worcester

This series of textbooks is aimed at students on Health and Social Care Foundation Degree programmes in FE and HE institutions. However, the books also provide short introductions to key topics for Common Foundation Programme modules and will be suitable for first-year undergraduate courses in a variety of Health and Social Care subject areas. Books in the series will also be useful for those returning to practice and for overseas nursing students. The series includes three types of textbook:

- Knowledge and Skills books;
- Theory and Practice books;
- Specialist books that cover specific professions, topics and issues.

All titles in the series will address the common elements articulated in relevant sector skill frameworks such as, for example, Skills for Care, Skills for Health, the NHS Knowledge and Skills Framework and the Code of Practice for Social Care Workers.

Other new and forthcoming titles in the series include:
An Introduction to the Principles and Practice of Care by Peter Unwin
ISBN: 978 1 906052 03 4

Understanding Research and Evidence-based Practice
by Bruce Lindsay
ISBN 978 1 906052 01 0

Values for Care Practice by Sue Cuthbert and Jan Quallington
ISBN. 978 1 906052 03 8

Communication and Interpersonal Skills by Elaine Donnelly and
Lindsey Neville
ISBN: 978 1 906052 06 5

Safe and Clean Care: Infection Prevention and Control for Health and Social Care Students by Tina Tilmouth with Simon Tilmouth
ISBN: 978 1 906052 08 9

Work-based Learning and Practice Placement: A Textbook for Health and Social Care Edited by Graham Brotherton and Steven Parker
ISBN: 978 1 906052 12 6

Visit **www.reflectpress.co.uk** for more details on these titles.

Introduction

Marjorie Lloyd and Peggy Murphy

> Education is the most powerful weapon which you can use to change the world.
>
> Nelson Mandela

WHO IS THIS BOOK FOR?

There is no doubt that the world is changing far too fast for many of us to keep pace. The only tool that we have to enable us to keep up with such change is our knowledge; knowledge that things are constantly changing but, also, that we can be influential in that change. Studying helps us to develop and expand our knowledge, which in turn helps us to learn how to adapt to change. The purpose of this book therefore is not simply to introduce students to study skills but to introduce them to learning how to learn. The skills presented in this book are not so unusual that no one has ever heard of them. Nor are they ideas that are unfamiliar to people who already implement them in their daily lives, whether or not they have attended university. Reflection, for example, is constantly cited as being a skill that everyone has but, perhaps, not everyone can use to the best of their ability.

This book is about helping students to develop learning skills so that they can get the best out of their time at university and enjoy the process of learning along the way. Learning should not be a chore but a discipline, something that we need to do each day to help us grow and survive modern living. Once learning becomes enjoyable we no longer need examinations, assignment deadlines or book lists to guide us, we set out on our own search for more knowledge and explore wherever the journey might take us. The intention of this book is therefore to demystify the process of learning in higher education so that students can actually get started upon their learning journey. So much valuable time is wasted trying to work out 'what the tutor wants' that the opportunity for gathering information and developing knowledge is lost. This book is for all those students who have asked us 'How many references do you want?', and who arrive at tutorials saying, 'I can't find anything to write about.'

We have attempted to address the issues that will help students from the beginning of their course up to graduate level, with some preparation for beyond graduation when they need to find a job with their newly developed skills and knowledge. The chapters address specific skills in order to help the student learn the skills that they need at a particular time and not bombard them with too much information all at once. If, as we suggest, learning is a lifelong activity, this book intends to help the student divide that learning into manageable chunks. The book is for students who are starting out on their learning journey and for some who have got a little lost along the way. It is also for the tutors of those students who patiently keep trying to steer them in the right direction.

HOW TO USE THIS BOOK

As experienced tutors, we have found little support from the literature in teaching students in higher education how to learn. This book is a response to the lack of support and we have given careful consideration to what are the essential study skills needed by the student during higher education study. The book will help students to prepare in advance for the transitional stages of learning in higher education when they and their tutor think they are ready to do so. There are some study skills books available that focus more deeply upon particular areas identified in this book but that involves the students having to buy many books to find the little bit of information that they need. This book provides brief but adequate information on the same study skills but in a version that is student-friendly, quick and easy to read. This is in recognition of the faster pace of student life and the fact that many students today are mature working parents who have little time and money to spare. The intention for this book is that the student uses it as a quick reference guide and reads each short chapter as and when required. Each chapter also provides student activities to support learning but, if time is short, these can be returned to later.

This book has been developed along the guidelines provided by the Quality Assurance Agency for Higher Education (QAA, 2001) *Framework for higher education qualifications in England, Wales and Northern Ireland* and the Quality Assurance Agency (QAA, 2006b) *Statement of common purpose for subject benchmark statements for the health and social care professions.* These guidelines provide a general outline of which study skills students should have achieved at certain stages in their academic development, alongside subject-specific skills that are part of everyday practice such as team-working and finding and presenting information. Often the skills discussed in this book are the hidden skills that are never shown but are nevertheless learned, usually the hard way. The QAA guidelines can be found in more detail in the Appendix of this book.

NAVIGATING YOUR WAY AROUND THE BOOK

The first few chapters focus on the main skills of finding information, referencing it correctly, writing skills for assignments and examinations, and learning styles. If students can develop these skills early in their undergraduate courses then they will be well prepared for what comes later.

The following chapters are to help the student make the transitional move from level 4 to level 5 which is approximately equivalent to a diploma level or basic/foundation degree. There will be greater demands made upon students who are studying at this level and they will need to learn how to study in groups, present their findings to others, gather information quickly; and learn from feedback from others including their tutors and their peers. This is especially important in vocational courses such as health and social care where these skills may also be included in professional competency requirements.

The final chapters help the student to develop their skills in preparing for the workplace and to develop their lifelong learning skills either through continued professional development or through higher education courses. Many universities use employability as a benchmark of the successful completion of an academic course. As the student comes to the end of this period of their study it is important that they are able to analyse their own skills and needs independently of others and be able to develop their skills towards whichever career path they have chosen to follow. Preparing students to 'fly solo' is an important part of the higher educational process, for which, again, it is difficult to find support from the literature. Students are expected to know what they want to do with the knowledge acquired. If they are not guided through this final transitional stage, they may fall by the wayside without a clear career path ahead of them. We believe that it is the role of the institution and the tutors within it to help the students prepare for their new lives with the skills they need to succeed. If we do not then all the hard work on behalf of the tutor and the student could be lost.

WHAT THIS BOOK CAN ACHIEVE

Essential Study Skills for Health and Social Care is intended for the novice student in higher education and for students who have difficulty developing the skills of studying. This may be because they have never been shown the way or because the information provided was not in the format that they required to understand it. We believe that the latter is the main reason for students not succeeding in their chosen area of study, which can have negative effects upon not only the student but also their families, their tutors and their peers. Education is an area of one's life where the only person you have to compete with is yourself and there is every reason to give yourself all the opportunity you can for success. While this book does not claim to tell you everything you need to know about learning to learn, it will provide enough basic information to get you started and keep you going. The rest, as they say, is up to you.

AUTHOR BIOGRAPHIES

Angela Hastings – Having worked in the field of midwifery and health visiting for 18 years in England and Wales, Angela is now a Senior Lecturer at Glyndŵr University in Wrexham. Most of her work involves teaching on the pre-registration bachelor of nursing programme. Angela has an interest in the student nurse experience of the use of the Welsh language in clinical practice and in the use of Web 2.0 technology to support teaching and learning.

Jessica Henderson – Jessica is Job Shop and Work Experience Officer at Glyndŵr University Careers Centre. This involves providing information, advice and suppport to students and graduates in finding and applying for jobs (CVs, application forms, interviews, etc.) and helping them find quality work experience opportunities. She also works closely with employers to source vacancies and work experience opportunities and to stay up to date with labour market information. Jessica is a member of AGCAS (Association of Graduate Careers Advisory Services), and NASES (National Association of Student Employment Services). She is currently studying for a Postgraduate Certificate in Careers Education, Information and Guidance in Higher Education.

Andrea Hilditch – Andrea is the Careers Information Officer at Glyndŵr University. Most of her work involves providing careers information for students and graduates; doing CV and application checks, providing interview preparation and mock interviews; facilitating group work sessions and presentations. She is currently studying for the Postgraduate Certificate in Careers Education, Information and Guidance in Higher Education and is a member of AGCAS.

Paul Jeorrett – Paul is the User Services Manager at Glyndŵr University. He is responsible for Library Services, the Health Centre and the Chaplaincy. Paul has worked as a professional librarian for 30 years, mostly in academic libraries, and has extensive experience of supporting students in their information needs and presentation skills. He is a regular presenter and facilitator at conferences and occasionally on community radio.

Liz Lefroy – Having worked in the fields of social care and education for 20 years, Liz is now a Lecturer at Glyndŵr University. She lectures on the BA social work course and has particular responsibility for enabling the participation of service users in all aspects of the course.

Marjorie Lloyd – Marjorie is a Senior Lecturer at Glyndŵr University. She co-ordinates the mental health branch pre-nursing programme and teaches post-qualifying practitioners in other courses. Majorie has worked in health and education for 20 years and has supported students in practical and academic study. Marjorie is currently studying at PhD level on empowering practice and is a Fellow of the Higher Education Academy.

Peggy Murphy – Peggy is a Senior Lecturer in health and is also admissions tutor at Glyndŵr University. Most of her work involves facilitating teaching and learning on the pre-registration Bachelor of Nursing course. She is currently studying for an MSc in professional education and is a Fellow of the Higher Education Academy.

Chris O'Grady – Chris is a Senior Lecturer at Glyndŵr University. Her main role involves co-ordinating the common foundation programme of the pre-registration Bachelor of Nursing course and teaching on the programme. Chris is a Fellow of the Higher Education Academy and is currently studying for an M.Phil.

Tracey Ross –Tracey Ross is a Senior Lecturer at Glyndŵr University and has a special interest in promoting critical reflection in clinical practice. Tracey teaches and supports students on post-qualifying courses in health and social care and is committed to continous professional development and lifelong learning. Her research area is concerned with the topic of human caring.

Nicola Watkinson – Nicola is Academic Liaison Co-ordinator at Glyndŵr University. Most of her work involves co-ordinating user education activities for staff and students on behalf of Glyndŵr University Library Service. She is a member of the Chartered Institute of Library and Information Professionals (CLIP) and a Fellow of the Higher Education Academy.

1

Literature Searching and Using the Internet Efficiently and Effectively

Nicola Watkinson

Learning outcomes

In this chapter you will learn how to:

- identify appropriate information sources, including electronic and internet sources;

- understand the principles of successful search strategies;

- identify tools to help you manage your information.

Scenario

Gill is preparing her first assignment for the end of the semester. She has been asked to write a 3 000-word assignment on reflective models and needs to find literature and references to support her assignment.

- Discuss the following chapter in class or with your tutor to clarify your own understanding.

Activity

Check your own learning needs and understanding by providing definitions for the following words/terms. The answers will become available as you read through the text.

Abstract, eBook, Internet Gateway, online database, URL

INTRODUCTION

During your studies, you will need to research and locate information to support your assignments. This is called a literature search. We will look at this process and examine it using traditional paper resources and then using the electronic, internet resources. Conducting a literature search can be a lengthy and complex process. However, taking a systematic approach, working through all your sources and keeping detailed records will make the process more manageable. The following guidelines should help.

SEARCHING THE LITERATURE – PAPER SOURCES

Plan/select topic

The key tip is to be organised! Some preliminary reading will be necessary. You need to check that there is enough literature on the subject that you intend to study. Use a library catalogue to gather items. You may find that too much has already been written to make it manageable. Formulate your ideas before starting the literature search. What are you trying to achieve?

Define the terminology

Break the main points of your assignment down into keywords and brainstorm if necessary. For each keyword, make a list of possible alternative words. Keep a list of the keywords that you intend to use. Dictionaries and thesauri (books containing lists of related words) may help you think of possible terms. Combine or remove these keywords to narrow or widen the scope of your search. Be general or specific depending on the number of results you get. Make a list of any acronyms (abbreviations), alternative spellings, related terms or synonyms (a word that means the same as another).

- An example of an acronym – NHS (National Health Service).
- An example of an alternative spelling – US *v.* UK spellings – pediatrician (US) or paediatrician (UK).
- Examples of related terms for 'listen to' – pay attention to, give advice, educate.
- Examples of synonyms – communication, conversation, confabulation, verbal intercourse, dialogue, debate, discourse.

This list may expand as you go along. You can return to sources to search them again with new terms and it is a good idea to keep a list of which terms you have used and where.

Define your parameters

Decide what limits you intend to impose on your search and stick to them. For example, are you only going to look at English language material? You may want to consider parameters for language, geography, time period, material type and sector.

Select your sources

You will need to consult different sources to find many types of information (some of these are listed later in this chapter).

Analyse references

References are sources of information or facts. Once you find a reference, you need to decide how useful it will be. Examine each reference critically and, for each one, ask yourself the following questions.

- Is it worth pursuing?
- Does it meet my defined parameters?
- Is it reliable?
- Is it unbiased?
- When was it published – are there more recent sources that I can use?
- What are the political views/social background of the author – is the author likely to be biased in some way?

Locate material

Once you have a list of references, you need to locate the material. You need to check to see if it is held in your local library or a library nearby. If not, you may wish to request it on an Inter Library Loan. There may be a small charge for this. Use any contacts you have – a colleague may well have a copy of something you are looking for. Organisations may be able to supply certain items.

Record information about the sources you find and use

It is important that you record details of your sources as you go along. This saves much time later on. Make sure that you have full references, including author(s), title, publisher, dates, page numbers, editions, volume number, part number, etc. Consider using a card index to help you keep track of what you have consulted and where. Copy useful quotes and keep the reference, including page numbers. You will need full references if you quote or refer to someone else's work. (See Chapter 2 for further information on referencing.)

If you have many results it may be worth downloading them into Reference Management software such as EndNote™, RefWorks™ or ProCite™. You can subscribe to this software as an individual or your library may hold a subscription.

Library catalogues

You can use your local university, college or public library to search for sources of information. You can often renew or reserve books via the OPAC (Online Public Access Catalogue), links to which are often available over the internet. Ask your library staff for details. You may be able to borrow materials from other libraries or, usually, at least photocopy materials within copyright restrictions. This usually means being able to copy up to 5 per cent or one complete chapter (whichever is the greater) from a book. You can also make good use of any libraries that you have access to if you are on placement, for example, NHS Trust libraries.

Keyword searching

While you are searching for items look for prominent authors in your field. What else have they written? If you do not find the items you want using a 'title' search try a 'keyword' search. Keyword searching looks for words in titles, subject headings and contents notes. It is the most flexible way of searching and is most useful if you wish to find items on a particular topic, with no prior knowledge of authors or titles.

eBooks

More and more books are being made available electronically. These are known as eBooks or electronic books. Services such as NetLibrary and MyiLibrary provide digital access to full-text books. You can search within the content of eBooks and your search terms are highlighted. Many eBook collections have links to online dictionaries if you are unsure of a term. There are often links to eBooks on many library catalogues. However, copyright is the same as for paper books.

Journals

Journals or periodicals are available in paper format or electronically through the internet. Most journals are published at regular intervals during the year and usually contain the most up-to-date information about a particular subject. As you study, it is important that you become acquainted with the current professional and specific journals such as the *Nursing Standard*, *Journal of Advanced Nursing* and the *British Journal of Social Work* that are relevant to your studies. Many journals allow their articles to be indexed and information from these indexes is often included in online databases, which will be discussed later in this chapter.

Research and government publications

Research and government publications include, for example, theses, reports, conference proceedings, government reports, enquiry findings. Many of these are available on the internet.

Statistics

Statistics can be gathered using the Office for National Statistics website (see the list of free internet sites beginning on page 17).

Organisations/professional bodies

These can be useful sources of information and often provide free literature and lists of publications. You can often join as a student and receive access to information. For example, Royal College of Nursing members can access the RCN E-library.

Reference collections

Many libraries have useful collections of materials including dictionaries, directories, encyclopaedias and yearbooks. Some reference books may be available electronically on the internet.

Library staff

Library staff are usually very helpful and a good source of information. Your library may also produce user guides and help sheets on various services to assist you.

SEARCHING THE LITERATURE – ELECTRONIC AND ONLINE SOURCES

Online databases

There are many online databases available to you as a student and many use similar search techniques. An online database enables you to search across different titles or just search one particular title. Some may give you the full article (full-text) and others may just give you references or an article abstract (summary). Many online databases are available on a subscription basis and you will be able to access these if your college or university has a subscription to that particular database (see Subscription sites below). However, you can also obtain a lot of quality information through free internet sites and we will look at these in detail later in this chapter. Useful online databases include the following.

Subscription sites

- **AMED (Allied & Complementary Medicine)** – AMED is produced by the British Library and covers a selection of journals in three separate subject areas: several professions allied to medicine; complementary medicine and palliative care.
- **BIOSIS** – life science information.
- **British Nursing Index** – a nursing and midwifery database, covering over 200 UK journals and other English language titles.
- **CINAHL** – Cumulative Index to Nursing and Allied Health Literature. CINAHL indexes over 2 900 journals from the fields of nursing and allied health. The database contains more than 1 000 000 records dating back to 1981.
- **Embase** – biomedical and pharmacological information.
- **IBSS (International Bibliography of the Social Sciences)** – the essential online bibliography for social science and interdisciplinary research.
- **Internurse.com** – this draws together articles from ten specialist journals including the *British Journal of Nursing*.
- **Journals@Ovid** – scientific, medical and academic research journals.
- **JSTOR** – important scholarly journals.

- **ProQuest Nursing Journals database** – full-text database for over 550 nursing-related publications from 1986 to the present.
- **PsycInfo** – a database of psychological literature from the 1800s to the present.
- **Royal College of Nursing (RCN)** – member access to full-text electronic journals via the RCN E-library.
- **Social Services Abstracts** – provides bibliographic coverage of current research focused on social work, human services and related areas, including social welfare, social policy and community development.

Please note that this list is not exhaustive and is for information purposes only. Check with your local library to see if they hold a subscription to a particular service.

Searching online databases

To access many online databases you will need a username and password, or your library may subscribe to the Athens or Shibboleth systems. Athens and Shibboleth are designed to simplify access to online databases with a single username and password. Ask your library staff for details.

Although they are usually different in content and coverage, most online databases use similar search processes and the following can be applied to many services.

- Use your keywords from your defined terminology. It is best to start with a basic search and you can usually search within keyword, title or author. You can combine your keywords in an advanced search and limit this by date of publication, author or journal. If you are unsure of how a keyword is spelt or you wish to search for several similar words you can use truncation and wildcards. Most databases use either '$' or '*' to do this. For example, to search for 'nurse', 'nurses', 'nursing' use the stem of the word 'nurs' and use nurs* to indicate to the online database that you have missed letters out at the end. Another example is, if you wish to search for articles that contain either the keyword 'woman' or 'women', using wom$n will search for both variations.
- You can also limit or refine within a search to narrow down your results. If you are satisfied with your search results many databases will allow you to save, download, e.mail or print your results. This means that you do not have to view your results on the screen but can save them to view at your leisure. This is usually known as 'marking' and is generally done by ticking a box to the side of each appropriate reference.

- Some online databases may only give you bibliographic details (title of article, journal in which this article appeared, author's name, page details, etc.) and some may give you just a summary or an abstract. You can often scan the abstract to see if the complete article is worth obtaining or not. You can photocopy the article if the journal is available in your library or you can obtain it via Inter Library Loan (see 'Locate Material' above).
- You can often save searches so that you can run them again at a later date. This will retrieve new articles about your chosen subject that have been published and indexed on that particular online database since your last search. You can often set up an e.mail alert service so you will be e.mailed articles that match your search criteria.

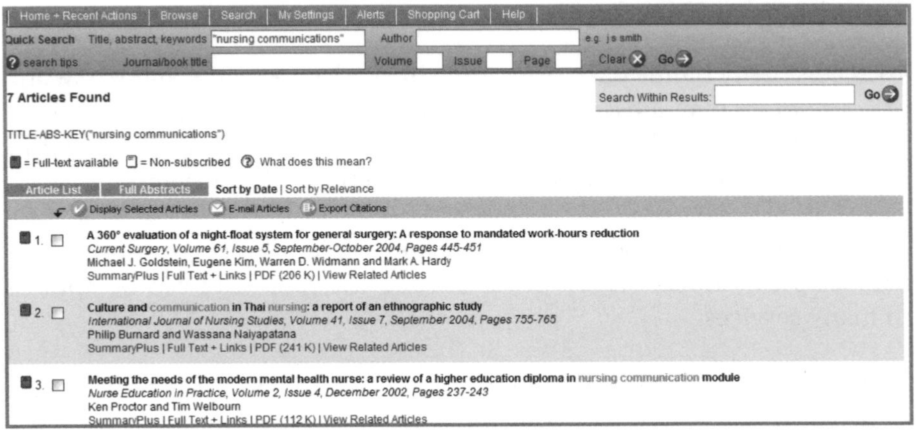

Figure 1 An example of online search results

Many articles that you do retrieve via online databases are in PDF or Portable Document Format. This enables you to search within the text of the article you have retrieved. You will need Adobe Acrobat installed on your computer to view PDF files. This is free to download from **www.adobe.com**, although Adobe Acrobat is often installed on university library computers.

For further help most online databases offer online help or your library may also produce guides on using various online databases.

The internet

The internet is a concept rather than a particular place. It is a collection of computers and computer networks, all linked with physical connections and special software. You can use the internet to exchange e.mail all over the world, to obtain software or to search for information. The World Wide Web (WWW) is a collection of internet sites and specially written pages, based on hypertext. Hypertext offers a means of moving from document to document within the World Wide Web. You will need a web browser on your computer to view the internet. The most popular browsers are Internet Explorer, Mozilla, Firefox, Safari, Opera and Netscape.

Web page URLs

A web page is constructed from text and graphic images and it can form links to other pages. Text that forms a link to another page appears in a different colour from the normal body of the text on that page. Graphic images can also be links. To locate a specific web page, you will usually need to know the address, or URL (Uniform or Universal Resource Locator). This is the address of a web page. URLs look like this: **www.rcn.org.uk** This is the URL for the home page of the Royal College of Nursing (RCN). Most URLs include a domain name. Some common domain names are as follows:

- .ac   academic (UK);
- .co   company;
- .com   commercial or company;
- .edu   educational (US);
- .gov   governmental;
- .org   non-profit organisation or charity.

If you do not have a particular URL, then you can do a subject or keyword search to find information using a search engine (see below).

If you go to the RCN's home page (**www.rcn.org.uk**) you will be able to see the URL in the white 'location' box at the top of the page. This location will change to display the current address of the page you are looking at as you search the internet. You can click in this box with your mouse and type in a new URL (this must be accurate) then press return to go directly to that page. If you receive an error message the site is either not available or you may have mistyped the URL.

Searching the internet

To search the internet there are a number of search engines available, such as Google (**www.google.co.uk**) and Ask (**http://uk.ask.com**). Search engines allow you to enter keywords in a box and then run a search to find sites that contain those words. You can use any of these search engines and, as you become familiar with searching, you can choose which one suits you best. Be as precise as you can with your search words; you are less likely to get misleading hits if you take time to think about what you are looking for. Try not to be too general to start with; you can always broaden your search later. In most search engines the '+' (plus) sign means that the word or phrase must appear in the documents retrieved. For example, if you type in elderly+vulnerable+financial+ abuse the search results will only include sites and pages that include these words.

You may need to use the scroll bar at the side of the page to move up and down within the search page. As your search is being executed, your browser's icon on the right-hand side of the toolbar will be moving. The search is not complete until the icon becomes still. Your search results will be displayed; usually ten hits at a time. If you want to view a particular site which is listed click on the hyperlink, which is usually the underlined title.

If you find a site which is particularly useful and which you may want to visit again, you can save it as a favourite for future reference. As you are viewing the page you want to save, go to 'Favourites' at the top of the screen, and down to 'Add favourites'. You can keep adding to this list. See also **del.icio.us** (page 20).

Saving and copying

The best way to save text is to highlight what you want by running the cursor over it. Select 'Copy' from the 'Edit' menu. Open Word and select 'Paste'. To save a page in HTML (Hypertext Markup Language) format select 'Save As' from the 'File' menu, insert either a floppy disk, CD, DVD or USB pen and select the drive to which you wish to save the file.

If you want to save an image, right click on the image and select the 'save image' option. Open up Word and go to the 'Insert' option on the toolbar. Select 'picture' and then 'from file'. Choose the image you have just saved and then click 'open'. The image should now appear on your document. If you want to resize the image, click on it and then, holding down the 'ctrl' button on the keyboard, use the mouse to move the corner of the image either further in or out, depending on whether you want to make it smaller or larger.

Useful internet sites

There are many other useful sites on the internet and a selection is given here. Free internet sites – health and social care related – include the following:

- **AgeInfo (www.cpa.org.uk/ageinfo/ageinfo2.html)** (accessed 2 June 2008) – an information service about old age and ageing provided by the Library and Information Service of the Centre for Policy on Ageing. Free restricted access only.
- **Bandolier (www.jr2.ox.ac.uk/Bandolier/index.html)** (accessed 2 June 2008) – a website about the use of evidence in health, healthcare and medicine. See also the National Library for Health.
- **BioMed Central (www.biomedcentral.com)** – 185 peer-reviewed open-access journals.
- **Centre for Reviews and Dissemination (www.york.ac.uk/inst/crd)** – reviews of research about the effects of interventions used in health and social care. Includes the Database of Abstracts of Reviews of Effects (DARE).
- **Cochrane Library (http://www.cochrane.org)** (accessed 2 June 2008) – high-quality independent evidence for health care decision-making. See also the National Library for Health.
- **Department of Health (www.dh.gov.uk/en/index.htm)** (accessed 2 June 2008) – provides health and social care policy, guidance and publications.
- **Institute for Public Policy Research (IPPR) (www.ippr.org.uk)** (accessed 2 June 2008) – research and innovative policy ideas for a just, democratic and sustainable world.
- **Medline (http://medline.cos.com)** (accessed 2 June 2008) – uses MeSH (Medical Subject Headings) which improve the accuracy of the search. See also PubMed.
- **National Library for Health (www.library.nhs.uk)** (accessed 2 June 2008) – a digital library for NHS staff, patients and the public that includes Bandolier and the Cochrane Library.
- **NICE** – National Institute for Health and Clinical Excellence **(www.nice.org.uk)** (accessed 2 June 2008) – an independent organisation responsible for providing national guidance on promoting good health and preventing and treating ill health.
- **PubMed (www.ncbi.nlm.nih.gov/sites/entrez)** (accessed 2 June 2008) – a service of the US National Library of Medicine that includes over 17 million citations (references) from Medline and other life science journals for biomedical articles back to the 1950s. PubMed includes links to full-text articles and other related resources.

- **Social Care Online (www.scie-socialcareonline.org.uk)** (accessed 2 June 2008) – the UK's most extensive free database of social care information includes research briefings, reports and government documents.
- **TRIP** – Turning Research into Practice **(www.tripdatabase.com)** (accessed 2 June 2008) – free evidence-based medicine site.

Please note that this list is not exhaustive and is for information purposes only.

Free internet sites – general:

- **Directgov (www.direct.gov.uk/en/index.htm)** (accessed 2 June 2008) – public services all in one place.
- **Europa (http://europa.eu)** – gateway to the European Union.
- **Info4local (www.info4local.gov.uk)** (accessed 2 June 2008) – the one-stop information gateway for local public services. You can use this portal to get quick and easy access to the information you need from central government departments, agencies and public bodies.
- **Intute (www.intute.ac.uk)** (accessed 2 June 2008) – a free online service providing access to free high-quality internet resources. Areas include Intute: Health and Life Sciences and Intute: Social Sciences.
- **National Statistics Online (www.statistics.gov.uk)** (accessed 2 June 2008) – free access to data produced by the Office for National Statistics.
- **Statute Law Database** (SLD) **(www.statutelaw.gov.uk)** (accessed 2 June 2008) – primary legislation of the United Kingdom made available online.
- **zetoc (http://zetoc.mimas.ac.uk)** (accessed 2 June 2008) – access to the British Library's Electronic Table of Contents of around 20 000 current journals and around 16 000 conference proceedings published per year. Free to most UK higher and further education institutions.

Please note that this list is not exhaustive and is for information purposes only.

Sometimes links to these and other sites are available on your library web page. You may also want to look at the websites of appropriate organisations, professional bodies, charities, etc.

As there is so much information on the internet, some of it good and some of it bad, it is important that you develop effective search techniques. As a rule, information from Wikipedia should not be used unless you can validate the information from other (legitimate) sources. Internet gateways are available to help you search for quality and reliable internet sites. An internet gateway is an online directory or catalogue that selects and evaluates websites. Intute (**www.intute.ac.uk**) is one example of an internet gateway. You can save Intute records of interest by registering with MyIntute, which is available on Intute, and receive a weekly alert listing new records that match your search criteria.

Learn how to use the internet effectively and efficiently

Some basic tips include:

- be as precise as you can within your defined search parameters;
- use double quote marks around phrases, for example, "National Health Service";
- narrow your search if necessary by using AND to combine terms, for example diabetes AND nursing;
- to omit words use NOT, for example, diabetes insipidus NOT mellitus and use OR to find alternative terms, for example children's OR young people's rights;
- use Advanced Search option to restrict your search by date of publication, language used or domain;
- think about the three 'Ws' of websites – why was the site created, who created the site and when (or where) was it created? This will help you evaluate the quality and relevance of the site.

'Judge: web sites for health' is an excellent website. This site gives useful information on how to search the internet for health information and how to judge the websites you find – **www.judgehealth.org.uk** (Childs) (accessed 20 December 2007). Although Judge is aimed at health consumers it has tips that are useful for everyone. Other sites of use are Intute: virtual training suite (**www.vts.intute.ac.uk**) (accessed 2 June 2008) which provides free tutorials to help you learn how to get the best from the web for your education and research and 'Internet Detective' (**www.vts.intute.ac.uk/detective**) (accessed 2 June 2008), which is a free online tutorial that will help you develop internet research skills for your university and college work. There are tutorials for Health and Social Care and Nursing, Midwifery and Health Visiting.

Internet tools

There are several tools that you can use to manage your internet searches:

- Saving bookmarks or favourites, such as del.icio.us;
- Using RSS feeds.

Del.icio.us (http://del.icio.us) (accessed 2 June 2008) enables you to store your internet bookmarks or favourites online, which allows you to access the same bookmarks from any computer and add bookmarks from anywhere too. You can also use del.icio.us to see the interesting links that your friends and other people bookmark and share links with them in return.

Many online databases have RSS – Really Simple Syndication or Rich Site Summary – summaries of new content or resources which enable you to keep up to date with new developments. For example, the National Library for Health (**www.library.nhs.uk/rss/Directory**) (accessed 2 June 2008) and Department of Health (**www.dh.gov.uk**) (accessed 2 June 2008) have RSS.

Activity – Revision Questions

1. What is a synonym?

2. How would you limit a search?

3. In addition to printing, in what other ways can you save search results?

4. What is a URL?

5. In addition to books and journals, where else can you search for information?

6. What is a domain (ac.uk, org.uk, gov.uk)?

CONCLUSION

Although literature searching can be time consuming it is worth learning correct techniques as it makes the process easier and less stressful. Do not get discouraged if you run into difficulties. You can ask for help or take a break and return to your work at a more convenient time.

Chapter summary

- Finding your way around the internet becomes easier with practice;

- Some tools will help you find appropriate information quickly;

- Keywords are useful in limiting/defining your search;

- Different domains will present you with different information.

2

Referencing, Plagiarism and Copyright

Marjorie Lloyd and Peggy Murphy

Learning outcomes

In this chapter you will learn how to:

- identify sources of information that you want to refer to within an assignment;
- accurately present references within the text of an assignment;
- accurately present quotations within the text of an assignment;
- compile a reference list and/or bibliography at the end of an assignment;
- avoid plagiarism and comply with copyright law.

Scenario

Sally was preparing her first assignment for the end of semester. She had been asked to write a 3 000-word assignment on communication skills. Sally had never written an assignment before as she had previously studied under the National Vocational Qualifications (NVQ) course. Although she had demonstrated all of her competencies this did not involve a great deal of writing. Sally was great at putting together a portfolio and had been helping fellow students with theirs but now she needed help with her assignment and was becoming very worried.

- How would you explain referencing to Sally? Discuss the following chapter in class or with your tutor to clarify your own understanding.

INTRODUCTION

The Quality Assurance in Higher Education Association (QAA, 2006a) advise that students should be provided with information from the organisation in which they are studying about how to support their work from the literature without breaking any laws. As part of any course undertaken, but especially within professional courses, you will be required to write an essay, project, assignment, dissertation or thesis for a degree. Therefore, you will frequently need to refer to literature that you have read in order to support an argument, illustrate a point or outline a particular theory (Maslin-Prothero, 2005). You must not, however, present another writer's materials or ideas without acknowledging where the information has come from. Failing to acknowledge the source of the information is termed plagiarism and carries serious consequences. Plagiarised work is usually disqualified and it can result in disciplinary action being taken (Proctor, 2006). It is unfortunate that many cases of plagiarism result from poor attention to detail, rather than any deliberate attempt to steal another's ideas.

Referencing literature is necessary for the following reasons:

- to prove that you have researched your topic and that your ideas have been presented in the light of published material;
- to substantiate your ideas and arguments;
- to acknowledge the source of your information and development of your ideas;
- to distinguish between your own opinions and those of others;
- to enable your readers to locate the source of the ideas that you have presented in order to study the material for themselves.

Activity

Check your own learning needs and understanding by providing definitions for the following words. The answers will become available as you read through this chapter:

In text referencing, Secondary referencing, Reference list, Bibliography, *Et alia*, Plagiarism, Paraphrasing, Copyright, Flagging, Quotation, Uniform Resource Locator, Harvard method.

METHODS OF REFERENCING

There are a number of different referencing systems (Rose, 2001; Mason-Whitehead and Mason, 2008). These include:

- the British Standard referencing system (which uses numbers to identify a writer's ideas);
- the Vancouver system (which also employs numbers that relate to the list at the back of the work) and
- the Harvard system, which uses the author's surname and date in the text and is the most popular system with British-based publishers.

Burnard (2004) suggests that the Harvard, or 'Name and Date', method of referencing is one of the most commonly used. However, you must check whether this system is used within the institution in which you are studying. The Harvard system has many variations so find out exactly how your institution requests that you reference your work (this is commonly stated in your student handbook).

There are two main aspects to the Harvard system. Firstly, a small reference or 'flag' is entered, in brackets, in the main body of your text at the point at which you make use of another writer's work. Secondly, a list, entitled 'References', is provided at the end of your work in which fuller details of all the references you have flagged are presented alphabetically. The purpose of this method is to ensure that the main body of your text is not cluttered up with large amounts of information, which may distract the reader. Sometimes students may become confused by the difference between a reference list and a bibliography. The difference is that a bibliography provides a list of sources read but not referenced or 'flagged' within the main text. In a reference system the text flags contain the minimum amount of information possible – just sufficient to locate the reference in the reference list at the end of your work.

Flagging references in your text

The flag is usually presented in the following form: a set of brackets containing the surname of the author to whom you are referring followed by the year of publication of the source document. Therefore, if the author's name does not appear naturally in the sentence, ensure the surname of the author and date of publication are in brackets.

> **Example**
>
> The flag in the text (please note all of the examples are fictitious):
>
> The original conclusions (Williams, 1990) have now been questioned (Reynolds, 1994).

> **Example**
>
> The full reference for the reference list at the end of your work:
>
> Reynolds, J. (1994) *Working at Communication*. Basingstoke: Palgrave
> Williams, P. (1990) *The Art of Communication*. London: Open University Press

If the author's name appears naturally in the text, add only the date in brackets.

> **Example**
>
> The original conclusions have now been questioned by both Reynolds (1994) and Roberts (1995).

Where a publication has been written by two authors, both should be acknowledged.

> **Example**
>
> A more recent study (Williams and Reynolds, 1996) disproved the earlier findings.

If there are three or more authors, only the first should appear in the text, followed by the term *'et al.'* (a shortened version of *'et alia'*, the Latin for 'and others').

Example

The flag in the text:

In a recent report, Smith *et al.* (1996) have* suggested yet another solution.

(*note the use of the plural for 'Smith *et al.*'). In the reference list at the end, you must ensure that the names of all of the authors are identified.

Example for the reference list at the end of your work:

Smith, J., Allwaring, P.M. and Watson, W. (1996) *The Modern Social Worker.* London: Piety Press Ltd

---

Secondary referencing

Sometimes it is impossible to go back to the original source to find an author directly. This can happen when an author quotes another author's work. You may want to use this information as a secondary reference source. In this case, the term 'cited in' must be used within the assignment.

Example

The flag in the text:

According to Murphy and Shepherd (1991, cited by Phelan and Bell, 2002), goals may be either short term or long term.

There are a number of ways of recording this at the back of your work, but one acceptable way is:

Murphy, P. and Shepherd, R. (1991) *Prioritising Workload.* Oxford: OU Press. Cited in Phelan, G. and Bell, Y. (2002) *Creating a Good Work/Life Balance.* Toronto: Positive Life Publishers

---

Wherever possible it is best to avoid this type of citation. Always attempt to go back to the original source of the information.

Referencing quotations

Quotations may be classed as direct or indirect. A direct quotation is when you extract a key word or a sentence from a source and do not alter it. When direct quotations are used, a page number must always accompany that quote in the text and in the reference list. If your quotation is less than two lines long, you should include it in your text in inverted commas.

Example

According to Aggleton and Chalmers, (2002, p. 70) 'once nursing problems have been identified, the nurse devises a care plan'.

Remember to add Aggleton and Chalmers' full details (including the page number) to your reference list at the end, as shown earlier.

If your quotation is longer than two lines, indent the whole quotation as a new paragraph, reduce the font to size 10 and use single line spacing (if you have been using double spacing in your main text). For quotations longer than two lines, you do not need to use inverted commas. Add the page number where the quote is taken from and use three full stops to indicate any word(s) you have missed out.

Example

Many academics have pointed out the need to develop writing skills in students. Newby (1989) asserts:

> Writing is like talking: a natural ability – once you have learned to do it. It develops with use in the right environment. You can learn how to write better . . . don't give up hope: the chances are that you can still improve considerably. (p. 5)

Remember to add Newby's full details to the reference list.

The use of direct quotations in work that you are submitting for assessment should be fairly limited. It only really makes sense to use a quotation where the words, or the phraseology, of the original author convey the meaning in an exceptional or memorable way. Broadly speaking, you should use your own words whenever possible to describe or explain the work of others. Any carefully selected quotes that you choose should be no longer than three or four lines. Avoid using too many quotations overall. As a guide, no more than 5 per cent of the total word count of your work should be made up of direct quotations.

Indirect quotations

This is when you refer to an extract but then put it into your own words (paraphrasing).

Example

Nurses, like other health care professionals, work with vulnerable people in situations that require them to communicate trustworthiness (Burnard, 2005). To facilitate this process they must be aware of how to communicate dependability to the people they are working with.

Alternatively, the same evidence could be referenced as follows:

Burnard (2005) states that nurses and health care professionals need to be aware of their unique position as patients/service users need to be able to trust them. The ability to do this involves being conscious of how to convey trustworthiness.

Then remember to put Burnard's (2005) entire reference in the reference list at the end, like so:

Burnard, P. (2005) *Counselling Skills For Health Professionals* (4th Ed). Cheltenham: Nelson Thornes

---

In general, make use of paraphrasing or précis as much as possible. This will best demonstrate your own understanding of the issues involved. Remember that you still need to acknowledge the sources of your ideas by citing references even when paraphrasing the work of others. Not to do so would be plagiarism.

The reference list

Your list of references appears alphabetically by author at the end of your document. In the Harvard referencing method, you must not use bullet points or numbers to identify each reference. The information provided for each reference must comply with a strict set of requirements that would enable any reader to locate precisely the items to which you refer.

There are many sources of information that must be referenced in slightly different ways so it is important to become familiar with the different requirements. The format of the reference will vary slightly according to the type of material to which it relates. You should note that the punctuation used and the emphasis given to sections of the reference is of great importance. For instance, the use of italics or bold or underlined text where specified is essential because it will help readers to identify the type of source material (for example, a book or a journal). The formatting information for different types of reference source is described below. One point to note is that a reference list includes the names of all authors of a source, no matter how many, and the term '*et al.*' must not be used in the final reference list.

Format for referencing books

- Name(s) of author/s, editor/s or the institution that has produced the book.
- The year of publication in brackets.
- The title of the book in italics (or bold text or underlined text if that is what your institution requires).
- The edition, if it is not the first edition.
- The place of publication.
- The publisher's name.

Note: the source of the information is highlighted in either bold, italics or underline. You must be consistent whichever way you choose to do this. In this example, the sources are books and are highlighted (in this case in italics).

Example

Carnall, C.A. (1999) *Managing Change in Organisations* (3rd Ed). London: Prentice Hall

Rudestam, K.E. and Newton, R.R. (2005) *Surviving your Dissertation: A comprehensive guide to content and process*. London: Sage Publications

---

For different books published in the same year by the same author, lower case letters are used to identify the different books in the flags in the text and in the full references at the end of your work:

Example

The flag in the text:

Dawson (1999b) employs more in depth interviews to support his earlier findings in Dawson (1999a), which suggested a link between stress and lack of leadership in the workplace.

Example for the reference list at the back of your work:

Dawson, R. (1999a) *The Politics of the Family*. London: Hugo Publications

Dawson, R. (1999b) *Working Women*. Oxford: Oxford University Press

---

Edited books should be cited under the editor's or editors' names and you include the term (Ed) or (Eds) in the reference:

Example

The flag in the text:

Lloyd and Murphy (2008) suggest that plagiarism is often due to a lack of understanding rather than simply flouting academic rules.

Example in the reference list at the back of your work:

Lloyd, M. and Murphy, P. (Eds) (2008) *Essential Study Skills for Health and Social Care*. Exeter: Reflect Press

---

Format for referencing authors of chapters

If you are directly quoting an author who has contributed to an edited book, cite the name of the author and the title of the chapter (in single inverted commas), the number of the chapter written by that author and then, following the word 'in', cite the referencing details of the source book.

Example

The flag in the text:

Hastings (2008) states the importance of preparation when attending an interview.

Example in reference list at the back of your work:

Hastings, A. (2008) 'CVs and interview techniques', Chapter 12 in Lloyd, M. and Murphy, P. (Eds) (2008) *Essential Study Skills for Health and Social Care*. Exeter: Reflect Press

---

Referencing journals

- Each author's name and initials.
- The year of publication in brackets.
- The title of the article in single inverted commas.
- The title of the journal, in italics (or bold or underlined text).
- The volume number.
- The issue number in brackets.
- The numbers of the first and last pages of the article.

Example

Weiner, B. (1985) 'An attributional theory of achievement, motivation and emotion'. *Psychological Review* Vol. 92, (12), pp. 548–73

Note the distinguishing difference between the format for referencing books and journals. With the former, it is the name of the book that appears in italics, bold or underlined text. With journals, it is the title of the journal because it is the journal that is the source of the article. Note also that you should use a consistent style in your choice of either italics, bold or underlined text for the journal title.

Referencing government publications

These are usually part of corporate authorship and should be listed according to the department responsible for publication. However, the citation should always commence with the words 'Great Britain'.

Example

Great Britain Home Office (1990) *The Hillsborough Stadium, 15 April 1989*: inquiry by Lord Chief Justice Taylor: final report. London: HMSO

Referencing research reports

If possible, it is important to include the subtitle and series information of the report.

- Author's name.
- Date of publication in brackets.
- Title and subtitle (if any) in italics (or bold or underlined).
- Research report number.
- Place of publication (if known).
- Publisher.

Example

BRESCSU, Building Research Establishment (1996) *Drawing a winner: energy efficient design of sports centre*. Good practice guide no. 211. London: Department of the Environment

---

Referencing internet sources

Remember that one of the purposes of referencing is to enable others to locate the original source of your ideas. As we all know, many internet sources are 'here today and gone tomorrow' and therefore, as a general rule, it is wise only to use internet references from reputable sources. Examples of reputable sources would include the Welsh Assembly

Government and the Nursing and Midwifery Council (Place *et al.*, 2006).

There is not, as yet, a standard related to referencing internet sources due to the rapid development of the internet. However, for credible internet sources you should follow the general rules for the referencing of material from other sources.

- Name of author(s) or institution that has produced the material.
- Year that the material or web page was produced in brackets (this is often at the very bottom of the web page).
- Title of the web page.
- The publisher of the website/page.
- The Uniform Resource Locator (URL) – this is the full web page address and usually begins with **http://**. The URL must be accurate, as any slight inaccuracies will prevent the reader accessing the information that you have referred to. An example of a URL is highlighted by the arrow in Figure 1, below:

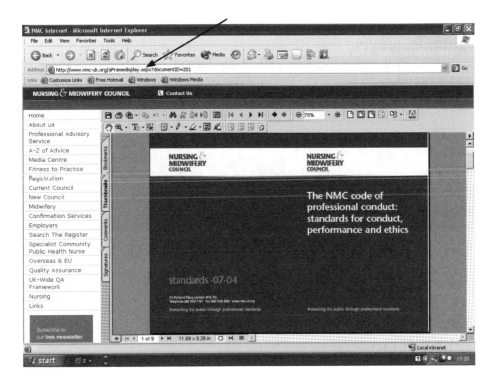

Figure 1 An example of where to find the URL on a web page

Please note that you must remember to include the date that the web page was accessed in brackets at the end of the reference.

Example

Nursing and Midwifery Council (2004) 'The NMC code of professional conduct: standards for conduct, performance and ethics' **http://www.nmc-uk.org/aFramedisplay.aspx?documentID= 201** (Accessed 28 July 2006)

Watson, J. (2006) 'Transpersonal caring and the caring moment defined'. School of Nursing, University of Colorado **http:// www2.uchsc.edu/son/caring/content/transpersonal.asp** (Accessed 29 July 2006)

Please note that the web page address is in bold as this is the source of the information (and it makes the URL easier to read).

Further examples of how to reference internet sources can be found in most of the reputable journals such as the *Journal of Advanced Nursing*. It is good practice to print off a copy of the web page you are referring to, if it is likely to be updated, as you may need to produce the evidence that you accessed the web page on the date that you have specified.

Referencing web sources in the text

If you are referring to one of the above internet referencing examples in the main text of a piece of work, do not reference the website. All you need to identify, as with a book or journal, is the surname of the author or the institution followed by the year. Refer to the guidance on the in text referencing of books or journal articles above.

Example

According to the NMC (2004), registered nurses must keep their skills and knowledge up to date.

Then remember to ensure that the NMC (2004) website reference features in the reference list.

Lecture notes and personal communication

It is not considered best practice to reference lecture notes and/or personal communication such as an e.mail. However, personal communication can appear in published writing when the author wants to demonstrate that they have discussed an idea or concept with someone in great depth and that discussion has influenced the course of the assignment. The above referencing guidelines should be applied to these sources and the general rules still apply that sources should, wherever possible, be obtainable by others. For example, name, date and time should, at the very least, be included in the reference, as should details of where the information can be found or evidenced. If a virtual learning environment is used to deposit lecture notes then this may be included in the references and you should state the course name and module title.

COPYRIGHT LAW

It is important to remember, when photocopying, scanning or using diagrams and pictures from other people's work, that these sources must be referenced properly. This might also include an adaptation from different sources or a direct copy. Publishing etiquette and UK copyright law establish that you should always seek permission from the original author and publisher to use other people's work, such as a picture or diagram, or you could be accused of breaking copyright law (UK©CS, 2004). However, a new copyright licence has been added to internet sources in particular that allows copying of any material without permission as long as it is not changed in any way and the author is recognised within normal referencing guidelines. Creative Commons Licences™ provide this service free to people who wish to upload pictures or text to the internet and allows people to use their material without breaking copyright law (Carvin, 2004).

REFERENCING QUIZ

Test your own knowledge with this referencing quiz.

1. What is it called when you do not acknowledge someone else's work and pass it off as your own?

2. Give three reasons why it is useful to provide references in your work.

3. What is the other name of the Name and Date referencing system?

4. When there is a single author, what information is included in the text of your essay (not in the list at the back of your work)? Choose one answer from the list below:
   a) the surname of the author;
   b) the surname and initial of the author;
   c) the surname of the author and the year of publication;
   d) the title of the publication and its date.

5. When do you put just the date in brackets – for example Murphy (2007)? Choose one of the answers below:
   a) at the end of a sentence;
   b) when the author's name appears naturally in the text;
   c) in every reference throughout the essay;
   d) alternately throughout the text.

6. When there are two authors – for example, Murphy and Jones, 2007 – how is this referenced in the text? Choose one of the answers below:
   a) Murphy and Jones (2007);
      or
   b) Murphy *et al.* (2007).

7. When using a secondary reference, how is this acknowledged? For example, you have read in Aggleton and Chalmers' (2002) work that they have referenced another text with two authors (Roy and Andrews, 1991), who have made an interesting point. How do you cite this in your text? Choose one of the answers below:
   a) Roy and Andrews (1991, cited in Aggleton and Chalmers, 2002);
      or
   b) Roy and Andrews (1991).

Please state whether the following statements are true or false.

8. A direct quotation is when you extract a key word or a sentence from a source and do not alter it.
   a) True.
   b) False.

9. When direct quotations are used, a page number must always accompany that quote in the text and in the reference list.
   a) True.
   b) False.

10. If your quotation is less than two lines long, you should include it in your text in inverted commas.
    a) True.
    b) False.

11. If your quotation is longer than two lines, indent the whole quotation as a new paragraph, reduce the font to size 10 and use single line spacing.
    a) True.
    b) False.

12. In general, make use of paraphrasing as much as possible. This demonstrates your own understanding of the issues involved and is better than just including direct quotes.
    a) True.
    b) False.

13. You still need to acknowledge the sources of your ideas by citing references even when paraphrasing the work of others. Not to do so would be plagiarism.
    a) True.
    b) False.

14. Your list of references appears alphabetically by author at the end of your document.
    a) True.
    b) False.

15. When referencing books, the following need to be included:
    - the name(s) of author(s), editor(s) or the institution that has produced the book;
    - the year of publication in brackets;
    - the title of the book in *italics*, or **bold** text or <u>underlined</u> text;
    - the edition, if it is not the first edition;
    - the place of publication;
    - the publisher's name.

Based on this information, spot the deliberate mistakes in the following reference list.

Rudestam and Newton (2005) <u>Surviving your Dissertation: A comprehensive guide to content and process</u>. Sage publications

Carnall, C.A. **Managing Change in Organisations** (3rd Ed) London:

16. When referencing journals, the following need to be included in the reference list at the back:
    - each author's name and initials;
    - the year of publication in brackets;
    - the title of the article in single inverted commas;
    - the title of the journal, in *italics*, or **bold** or <u>underlined</u> text;
    - the volume number;
    - the issue number in brackets;
    - the date of publication;
    - the numbers of the first and last pages of the article.

Based on this information, spot the deliberate mistakes in the following reference of a journal.

Weiner (1985) '<u>An attributional theory of achievement, motivation and emotion</u>'. Psychological Review, Vol. 92, No.12.

3

Learning Styles and Problem-based Learning

Peggy Murphy

Learning outcomes

At the end of this chapter you will be able to:

- define learning, learning styles and problem-based learning;

- understand the introduction to Kolb's (1984) experiential learning cycle;

- identify different types of learning styles;

- use the knowledge about your individual learning style to improve your learning experience;

- discuss the advantages and disadvantages of problem-based learning.

WHAT IS LEARNING?

Activity

Take a few minutes to answer the question 'What is learning?'

Definition of learning

Historically, teaching implied the active giving of knowledge. Therefore, learners were the passive recipients of knowledge (Fry *et al.*, 2003).

However, this division in the roles of teacher and learner is now recognised as artificial. Teaching – and learning – is documented as a two-way process where both student and tutor are jointly occupied in the pursuit and acquisition of knowledge. According to DeYoung (2003) the definition of learning is dependent upon the theoretical stance from which you view it. The behaviourist approach perceives learning as the acquisition of both knowledge and skills that cause a change in the person's behaviour. The cognitive approach is more concerned with what sense and meaning a person gives to new knowledge, rather than simply focusing on a change in behaviour (DeYoung, 2003). In general learning involves some sort of transfer of knowledge or skill; it takes place when people who were once novices become more expert (Benner, 2001). According to Cottrell (1999, p. 42) learning has occurred when there is sufficient understanding that a person can 'explain, teach or demonstrate it to others'.

Activity

Write down any factors that help you to learn. For example, do you listen to music when you revise or prefer silence? Do you study better with someone to bounce ideas off or do you prefer to learn alone? Do you prefer encouragement from tutors or do you need a metaphorical 'kick' to motivate you?

Activity

Identify any factors that have hindered your learning: for example, being frightened of making a fool of yourself; or physical problems such as poor hearing; or emotional blocks such as not feeling good enough.

Definition of learning styles

Learning styles describe the way in which people observe, conceptualise and recollect information. When learning improves so does a person's self-esteem (which has a further impact upon their learning). This is part of the cycle of learning. Understanding how to help students succeed in their learning is central to good education.

When you buy a new mobile phone do you read the instruction manual first to find out how it works or do you just press buttons until you find out by trial and error? Have you ever attended a lecture on a subject that appeared at the time to be way over your head, only to have it explained in a different manner later and be able to fully grasp the concept? This happens because people learn in different ways (DeYoung, 2003; Cottrell, 1999). We approach learning from different directions. Some prefer to study alone, others enjoy learning in groups. Some learn best from applying theoretical notions to practical settings, others learn best from actual experience. The term 'learning style' has been popular since the 1970s, often used interchangeably with the term 'cognitive style' (DeYoung, 2003). DeYoung (2003, p. 31) defines learning style as '. . . the habitual manner in which learners receive and perceive information, process it, understand it, value it, and recall it'.

The main point of knowing about learning styles is that when you understand how you learn you can plan how best to use your time. In other words, once you become aware of your preferred learning style you can use this information to help you to work smarter rather than harder. Being aware of your learning style helps you take some control; you can decide which learning activities suit you best and thus you can increase your learning potential. You do not always have to work harder to achieve the best results. When you know the way that you learn best, you can avoid continuously making the same mistakes. For example, if you know you rush in and always offer your suggestions first in group work, then you can make a deliberate decision to stand back at the next opportunity and let someone else offer their opinion while you give yourself time to reflect and consider their views (DeYoung, 2003).

The theory of Experiential Learning

Kolb (1984) wrote about experiential learning and devised a four-stage model (see Figure 1). He proposed that learning starts with 'concrete experience' (or being involved in a new experience) and then during the next stage the person 'observes and reflects'. They can do this by watching others or by reflecting upon their own behaviour within the new experience. From this, the person moves on to stage three whereby they develop ideas or 'abstract theories' on how this new knowledge can be put to use. Finally the person 'actively experiments', which means that they use their new knowledge to make decisions and solve problems (DeYoung, 2003).

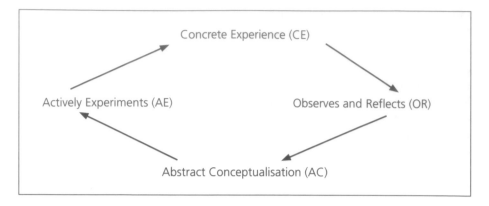

Figure 1 Kolb's four-stage model of experiential learning

The emphasis of his theory is on learning as a process rather than an outcome. Kolb (1984) proposed that there were two main modes of learning or continuums. He said that most people learn through either thinking or feeling (DeYoung, 2003), arguing that this occurs from either concrete experience or abstract conceptualisation. Kolb acknowledged that people tend to learn better one way rather than another and that this results in a unique learning style for each person. Kolb (1984) identified four learning styles based on this concept. He named them the converger, the diverger, the accommodator and the assimilator.

The converger

The converger is a person who learns by both concrete experience (CE) and abstract conceptualisation (AC). This person is a problem solver and often tends to work in technical environments rather than with people.

The diverger

The diverger is one who learns best from concrete experience (CE) and reflective observation. This type of learner has a good imagination and is a 'touchy, feely type'. This learner is people-oriented and works well in groups.

The accommodator

The accommodator also learns best from concrete experience (CE) but enjoys active experimentation (AE) as well. This type of person likes to 'task and finish'. This person solves problems by utilising a trial and error approach and can be a risk taker.

The assimilator

The assimilator emphasises abstract conceptualisation (AC) and reflective observation (RO). This learner can use inductive reasoning and create theoretical models. People who have this learning style prefer playing with ideas rather than putting them into practice.

Kolb (1984) viewed learning as a fluid process that moulds and remoulds students throughout life. He proposed that people are more prone towards a certain learning type or learning style, and that gravitation to this particular style is based on past experience, heredity and environmental demands (Kolb, 1984; DeYoung, 2003). Honey and Mumford (2006) based their work on learning styles on Kolb's (1984) principles. They described the four major learning styles as Activists, Reflectors, Theorists and Pragmatists.

Activists

These learners throw themselves in at the deep end to immerse themselves fully in any new experience. They enjoy living in the present. They are good at brainstorming any problems they are set. Activists enjoy being challenged academically but, as much as they enjoy problem solving, they can find implementing strategies tedious. They are often outgoing people but can be self-absorbed and allow themselves to be dominated by new experiences. They are good at leading others in both problem solving and role-play.

Reflectors

This type of learner likes to take a step back and consider problems from a range of perspectives. They like to gather all of the information and analyse it thoroughly before coming to a conclusion. They appear cautious and can leave others to lead while they take a back seat. They have the ability to think about the wider picture and are tolerant of the views of others. They are generally good at projects that do not have tight deadlines.

Theorists

These learners adapt anything they have observed to create logical arguments. They think about problems methodically in a vertical, step-by-step way. They have the ability to assimilate differing facts into rational theories. They can also have uncompromising tendencies when working in a group and do not feel comfortable until things become more organised. These people enjoy analysing data and take pleasure in models. Theorists are good at understanding complex problems.

Pragmatists

Pragmatists like trying out new ideas and techniques to see how they work in practice. These learners like to experiment. They are keen to get on with work but they are often impatient (particularly in open-ended discussion). Although they are frequently the first to take the opportunity to try out new concepts, pragmatists are often sceptical until they can see how an idea 'fits' in practice. They learn best when there is an obvious link between the topic being studied and an existing need.

Figure 2 outlines the strengths and weaknesses of these four types of learner and describes the strategies they can employ to improve their learning.

Learning style	Strengths	Weaknesses	Strategies to improve learning
Activist	Flexible, unbiased, ready to have a go, optimistic about change.	Risk taker, takes too much on board, bores easily and can be impetuous.	Write a risk assessment for each project that you tackle.
Reflector	Careful, thorough and methodical, thoughtful, good listener, rarely jumps to conclusions, good at assimilating.	Reluctant to participate, can be slow to come to any conclusion, overcautious, not always assertive and can lack the ability to socialise easily.	Develop a time plan along with your essay plan. Work backwards from deadlines (see Chapter 8 on time management).
Theorist	Logical, rational and objective, good at researching, disciplined approach.	Restricted in lateral thinking, has difficulty with uncertainty, intolerant of subjective thought.	Read two newspapers from different political persuasions and write a comparative analysis of one article from each perspective.

Pragmatist	Practical and realistic, down to earth, keen to test things out, straight to the point	Can be disinterested in theory and principles, impatient with waffle, tendency to be task oriented.	Make opportunities to experiment. Write action plans with accompanying time frames.

Figure 2 Strengths, weaknesses and strategies to improve learning (Honey and Mumford, 2006)

Activity

Establishing your Learning Style

There are many online tests that you can do to ascertain your learning style. Honey and Mumford (2006) is one of the best known and is based upon Kolb's (1984) model. These are a few other websites you can visit to find your own learning style.

www.ldpride.net/learningstyles.MI.htm
(accessed 4 June 2008)
http://agelesslearner.com/assess/learningstyle.html
(accessed 4 June 2008)
www.learning-styles-online.com/inventory/
(accessed 4 June 2008)
**http://adulted.about.com/od/learningstylesqu/Learning_
Style_and_SelfAssessment_Tests.htm**
(accessed 4 June 2008)

Some other types of learning styles

There are many other types of learning styles. For example, holistic (global) thinkers have a desire to get the whole picture quickly; these people want an overview of broad categories before getting bogged down with the details. This method of thinking involves processing information simultaneously, rather than in a sequential manner. The natural preference of this type of learner is to make connections with any new information so that they can relate it to the things that they already know. This style of learner likes to see the big picture first (DeYoung, 2003). The drawback of this style is that the proponents have a desire to overgeneralise and often do this without supporting their assertions with sufficient evidence (Quinn, 2000). Countering this approach are the analytical thinkers. These people process the intricacies of details in a logical manner. They process information in an objective manner and do not need to relate new information to their personal values or previous experience. Quinn (2000) states that the negative aspect of this type of learning style is that the students tend to have difficulties in displaying an understanding of how the components interrelate and lack the ability to see an overview of the topic.

Those students with a verbal approach to learning represent knowledge in terms of words or verbal associations. Those with a visual approach remember better by using pictures or images. Quinn (2000) states that some students can employ both holistic and sequential learning approaches when appropriate; he names these learners 'versatile'. DeYoung (2003) reminds us that students rarely learn exclusively in one style and proposes, like Kolb (1984), that it may be advantageous to think of these approaches as continuums. What is evident is that no one is a completely holistic thinker or learns purely through the visual medium. The relevance of knowing about learning styles is simply that most of us incline towards a preferred way of learning. The challenge to lecturers is to ensure that they design teaching and learning activities to incorporate all learning styles. The challenge to students is not simply to learn from the style they feel most comfortable with, but also to adapt in order to learn from other equally valuable strategies.

Activity

Imagine you are the world's best student. How would you set about your work? Would you do anything differently from the way in which you study now?

INTRODUCTION TO PROBLEM-BASED LEARNING (ALSO KNOWN AS ENQUIRY-BASED LEARNING)

Health and social care professionals need to be knowledgeable but, more than this, they need to be wise. They need to be able to apply what they know so that they can help people manage problems in real-life situations. Applying knowledge includes problem solving but it also involves professionals' transferring their skills to patients/service users and clients to enable them to access knowledge for their own benefit. This is one strategy to assist patients and service users to empower themselves. Knowing your own style and respecting that other people have different learning preferences is important in order to accommodate everyone's learning needs. Awareness of this enables health and social care professionals to support service users and patients to investigate the issues that concern them. This process is enhanced when the teaching methods used match the preferred learning style of the patient/service user.

Many 'chalk and talk' lectures only stimulate comprehension and retention of information. Students on professional courses need to be able to analyse and apply information (Prosser and Trigwell, 2001). The skills that are required to problem solve include collecting information, analysing it and then being able to apply the knowledge (Price, 2003). Critical thinking and the ability to synthesise knowledge (which is the capacity to create new ideas from the information gathered from different sources by using reasoned principles) are significantly improved when students employ a problem-solving approach (Wilkie and Burns, 2003). Central to both health and social care is the ability to work with other team members from your own profession and with members of other professions in the multi-disciplinary team. Problem-based learning provides students with a dynamic way to learn how to interact with others in a safe environment.

What is problem-based learning?

Problem-based learning (PBL) is a teaching and learning strategy that involves setting students real-life scenarios that provide real-life problems in an attempt to encourage them to think for themselves and subsequently find their own solutions (DeYoung, 2003). Fry *et al.* (2003) suggest that this pedagogical approach involves a large amount of small group work based on sound educational reasoning. They propose that learning happens after students identify their learning needs following a 'trigger' scenario that includes the problem. This approach involves students co-operating and collaborating in groups to investigate a problem and then presenting their work back to the class for assessment and feedback by the tutor (Mason-Whitehead and Mason, 2008; Price, 2003). This type of exercise goes some way towards preparing students for the real world they will enter as professionals. It also helps give them the skills to become proficient lifelong learners. This technique grew from an increasing frustration with traditional teaching methods and in recognition that health and social care professionals are required to be skilled in independent lifelong learning. DeYoung (2003) stated that several studies have found PBL to be at least as effective as, or even more effective than, traditional methods. In addition to its being an effective learning strategy, research by Colliver (2000) found that students reported that learning by PBL is more motivational and that many find this method more enjoyable than traditional methods.

Components of problem-based learning

Learning using this method involves both inductive and deductive reasoning. Students gather information to create theories about the situation and use these to establish whether they can resolve the situation (Price, 2003). Learning takes place in small groups in which students learn not only how to solve hypothetical problems but also how to cope with the difficulties of working with others (see Chapter 5, Learning in groups and teams). Learning to solve problems raises many issues such as emotions and confusion. Problem-based learning facilitators assist the group not only to complete the academic exercise but also to come to terms with every aspect of this method of learning. Problem-based learning has the following features.

- It provokes critical thought. Probing questions can be used by facilitators to encourage precise exploration of the situation to be studied.
- It utilises a variety of methods of enquiry.
- Learning recognises that problems in the real world reflect that life is a 'messy business' and that, as a result of this, there are no perfect solutions (though some work better than others).
- Although the group learns together, each member has responsibility for their own individual element.
- It encourages each member to test the information brought to them and to debate its value.
- It acknowledges each member's strengths and weaknesses.

Activity

1. Which groups do you belong to? For example, consider groups such as family, fellow students, work colleagues and interest groups.

2. How has your learning been shaped by being part of these groups?

Working in groups can enhance your knowledge considerably (see Chapter 5 for more information on working in groups). However, this method of working can also be fraught with problems. To minimise potential problems it is often beneficial for all members to consider working within an agreed framework. Ground rules are best observed when the suggestions come from the group members themselves.

Suggested ground rules for PBL groups

1. The group will nominate a chair and a secretary who will summarise what is to be considered and discuss what needs to be investigated. The chair's role is to welcome and encourage contributions from the group. At each session the chair and secretary may rotate in order to develop all members in these roles.
2. All members are to be present at each planned meeting. If a student cannot attend they need to inform the group secretary.
3. All of the exploratory work will be shared among the entire group.
4. Members are to listen, without interruption, to each member's feedback. Any questions will be addressed at the end of the member's presentation to the group.
5. Any challenges and evaluations made about the work presented need to be directed at the new information (not the group member who presents it). This is done in recognition that discussion is better when it is both honest and constructive.
6. The group will regularly review the analysis of the problem they are considering. If they come to a standoff they will seek guidance from the facilitator.
7. The facilitator's role is to act as the group's guide, not the boss.

The pros and cons of PBL

Problem-based learning assists students to understand how various subjects, such as biosciences and sociology, interrelate in a given situation. In many vocational courses, such as nursing and social work, skills are formally taught in the classroom. It is only when students are out in real placements that these skills can be put into practice. This can leave a 'learning hiatus', which expands the theory/practice gap. Problem-based learning offers a more seamless approach to learning with the aim of increasing students' understanding (Mason-Whitehead and Mason, 2008).

Another advantage of this type of learning method is that PBL can be used to teach an interprofessional learning course. That is, students from various professional courses (such as social workers, nurses and occupational therapists) can all work together in small groups to foster a climate of co-operation within the multi-disciplinary team (Fry *et al.*, 2003; Glen and Leiba, 2002). The theory behind interprofessional learning is that all of these professions will need to work together to provide care packages for people out in the real world. Problem-based learning provides an environment within the relative safety of a classroom setting in which it is possible to see how each of the health and social care professionals can work together for the benefit of the patient/service user.

Problem-based learning is more appropriately suited to small group teaching when there is a lot of time to discuss and debate any of the issues that arise. Experienced facilitators are aware of how to take a back seat and trust the students to establish the points to investigate; this is not always easy for less experienced tutors. This method of learning takes a lot of time and requires a high staff/student ratio. This type of work often highlights the non-contributory members of the group and can also suffer from any personality clashes within the group (Fry *et al.*, 2003). There are also resourcing implications with PBL as this approach to learning requires a large number of separate classrooms/study areas rather than a large lecture theatre (Fry *et al.*, 2003; Glen and Leiba, 2002).

One of the most important aspects of using PBL is that it gives students the confidence and ability to find things out by themselves then critique the information they have gathered. As PBL challenges students to become interactive in solving problems before they have been spoonfed the solution by lecturers, this process facilitates lifelong learning in a way that traditional methods do not (Wilkie and Burns, 2003). Problem-based learning encourages the students to develop their communication skills and contribute to their own development. It allows students to interact fully with their course and gives them permission to shape their own curriculum (Fry *et al.*, 2003; Prosser and Trigwell, 2001).

An example of a PBL scenario

Before commencing on a programme of study including PBL students should be introduced to the concept of this method of learning. It is also important to emphasise to the students that they are dealing with an authentic case history.

Scenario

A 28-year-old man has just been diagnosed with insulin dependent diabetes mellitus (IDDM). He and his wife have three young children, all under school age. He is the only wage earner in his family and has only just (two months ago) secured a full-time post working in the local chicken factory. He does not appear to have accepted his recent diagnosis and is reluctant to inject insulin or learn about how best to manage his condition. Using a holistic perspective, how would you help this man and his family come to terms with what has happened, and which members of the multi-disciplinary team do you need to liaise with in order to assist the man?

The students are placed in small groups to work on this issue. They can spend about an hour deciding how they will divide up the work and research the problem. The facilitator is present to guide the group. The students should not be 'given' the answers, as the objective of PBL is to solve a problem and not to be presented with the solution. The group facilitators, who are experts in the field, are often given a crib sheet by the PBL organiser with the salient issues to cover from the scenario. They can use this to steer the group if they start to deviate from the point. This is true education in a two-way process, as it is not unusual for the groups to offer pertinent suggestions that have not even been considered by the tutors.

The next session will be scheduled for approximately a week later to enable students to investigate the issue and bring their research to feed back to the group. This session will take about an hour (depending on the size of the group) and will allow for discussion around each student's material. Some PBL work involves the students finding out what happens to the patient/client or service user over a specific period and encourages them to think about how to address each of the issues in a sequential way. They await each week's 'episode' after feeding back their previous week's work.

Problem-based learning emerged to narrow the theory/practice gap. It has been put forward as a learning and teaching strategy that improves a student's analytical skills. It provides a relatively safe environment in which to make mistakes and put ideas into practice. This method encourages student participation, which in turn encourages students' learning at a deeper level. Although it has strengths and weaknesses, on the whole it is viewed by both students and lecturers as educationally worthwhile.

REVISION QUIZ

1. Give a definition of learning.

2. What are the four stages of Kolb's experiential learning model?

3. Which 'type' learns best through concrete experience – the accommodator, the converger, the diverger or the assimilator?

4. What type of learner are you?

5. Define problem-based learning (PBL).

6. How does PBL differ from traditional methods?

7. Name six aspects of learning this way.

8. Why have ground rules for PBL?

9. What are the main advantages of learning through PBL?

4

Writing Essays and Reports

Marjorie Lloyd

> When Higher Education contributes to the formation of complex achievements, it is contributing to people's futures, because these are achievements that are valued in professional life and citizenship.
>
> Knight, 2007, p. 74

Learning outcomes

At the end of this chapter you will be able to:

- plan the outline of a summative assignment or examination;
- develop your knowledge of the essay writing process;
- find information from a variety of reliable sources.

INTRODUCTION

It is not uncommon to feel nervous when you begin a course of study, with many unanswered questions running around in your mind. You are not alone but, if this is the first time anyone from your family or among your close friends has embarked upon higher education study, there will be no one for you to ask in the confidence that they will be sympathetic.

This chapter will help you answer some questions about how you can get the best out of your study time and enjoy the whole experience more. Some colleagues talk fondly of their student days being the best part of their lives and an enjoyable experience should be what you are also aiming for, not three years of anxious anticipation (QAA, 2006a). This chapter will address some of the anxieties common to many students such as:

- how do I write an assignment, exam essay or report?
- what do I include?
- what do I exclude?
- how do I find information?
- how do I know if the information is good enough?
- and – probably the most anxiety-provoking question – where do I begin?

This chapter will explore in more detail some of the skills you will need to develop in order to cope with the amount of work you are required to produce for your course of study. In addition, it will also provide you with an overview of the institutional requirements that guide all higher education courses in the United Kingdom, from the Quality Assurance Agency (QAA, 2001) as outlined in the Appendix at the back of the book. The QAA provide benchmark statements for many courses that are related to work-based qualifications, as well as the main academic levels of study from certificate to diploma and from foundation degree to honours degree, masters degree and doctorate programmes of study. The QAA are therefore quite influential alongside professional organisational bodies that require higher education institutions to meet their own standards of achievement. When your lecturers are preparing your courses and assessments, they are basing their requirements of your standard of achievement upon the standards required by these other professional bodies. This will be discussed in more detail later in this chapter but is acknowledged here to help you recognise the quality cycle that is in place around your academic study.

BEGIN AT THE BEGINNING

> In higher education 'assessment' describes any process that appraises the individual's knowledge, understanding abilities or skills.
>
> (QAA 2006a, p. 4)

Where to begin will depend upon what type of assessment you are expected to complete. There are many types of assessment such as written assignments, examinations, research reports, literature reviews, theoretical analysis, role-play and poster presentation but, for the purposes of this chapter, we will focus upon three main types – the written examination, report writing and the written assignment. All of these assessments, like most others, require a period of preparation and organisation. You may also be asked to submit work for these assessments either formatively or summatively. Formative work, such as a mock exam or poster presentation, is informally assessed, while summative work is given a mark that is fixed and unchangeable. Formative work assignments are not always taken seriously because the student knows that they are not being given a final mark. However, formative work is a good way of obtaining feedback from which you can actually improve your final or summative mark, so it is important to know the difference and the value of each. Although formative work is more informal, the feedback may be more important and useful than in summative assessments (QAA, 2006a).

Many tutors notice that students lack a systematic way of approaching their written work which, like any other activity, requires you to go through a series of steps to achieve a good outcome. For example, we learn to go through a number of steps to drive a car or it will not get us where we are trying to go. These steps become routine after a period of time but, to begin with, students may need a framework to help them. I developed the 'PROCESS Framework' of academic writing (Lloyd, 2007, p. 50) with those students in mind. The word 'process' in this context is an acronym for the steps or stages that are required to produce a robust piece of written work and they can be described as follows (Figure 1).

The PROCESS Framework of Academic Writing (adapted from Lloyd, 2007)	
Planning	What is it you are trying to achieve?
Referencing	How will you find out what you need to know?
Organisation	How will you collect your information together?
Composition	What level of understanding is required?
Engineering	How will you construct your assignment?
Spelling	How will you know that you have the correct terms?
Structure	How will you present/argue your findings?

Figure 1 The PROCESS Framework (adapted from Lloyd, 2007)

All of these stages will be discussed in more detail below. The framework will also provide the student and their tutor with an outline of what needs to be discussed within tutorial sessions. This helps both the student and the tutor become better prepared to get the most out of the time available, as most often students are limited to a certain number of meetings with their tutor.

MAKE A PLAN

Planning can be something you really do not think you have the time for but it will be invaluable to help you keep on track while you are becoming organised. Planning helps you to map out your initial ideas, which you can then share with a friend or your tutor who can help you keep on track. The more elaborate your plan is now the easier it will be to follow when you get nearer to your deadline. It is never too early to start planning. You will also need to think about how you are going to plan to deliver your assessment, which will improve the presentation when it is finished. These may seem simple suggestions now but in the anxiety and confusion of a looming deadline, they can help you to make sure you have remembered everything. For instance, have you thought about having:

- the right equipment;
- enough paper, ink cartridges and pens;
- enough time to complete and print out the finished document;
- enough books and resources, or access to resources such as library/ printing cards;
- a quiet space for studying/reading/thinking;
- a filing system for all the papers you will collect?

Some students create their own system of information storage but this tends to happen later on in the course when they have learned from their past mistakes. One third year student recently said to me, 'If only I'd known then what I know now', which of course is impossible but their hindsight can be extremely useful to new students. It may be helpful therefore to use your peers as a support system, talk to them over coffee about how they plan and organise their study. Some universities have buddy systems where more experienced students support students who have just begun a programme of study. This is not the same as plagiarism where students copy other students' work, knowingly or not. The buddy system simply helps you to find your way around and become organised quickly.

> **Activity**
>
> **Making a deadline checklist**
> Start writing yourself a deadline checklist, which you can add to your calendar or diary well in advance of the hand-in date. Discuss with your tutor if you think you are going to have any problems. They may be able to help you access support. Above all, don't just hope that the problem will go away – it probably won't.

Mind mapping

This activity can be carried out on a computer, using specific programmes, or on a piece of paper, whichever is more convenient for you to use. Whatever method you use, make sure you are comfortable using that particular method as you have no time for trying to find lost ideas when you start working on your assessment. This will only cause you further anxiety, which you do not need. You will have been given an assessment briefing, usually at the beginning of the module that you are currently studying, so will need to go back to the briefing to check what is required. There should at least be some learning outcomes like those at the beginning of this chapter, and maybe some further guidelines about presentation, etc. A mind map (see Figure 2), also sometimes known as a spider diagram, is a collection of associated words on a page with linking lines and words to connect them all together. Mind maps usually begin with a central word or idea – perhaps the exam or essay title – in the middle of the page and then spread out in a sort of loose spider's web of related words and ideas – as many as you can think of. Once you can no longer think of ideas that might be useful to your study, you can move on to the next stage of gathering information on aspects that you now know you want to write about. Don't worry about forgetting something important as you can always add it later; for now, you have a plan that you can start working on.

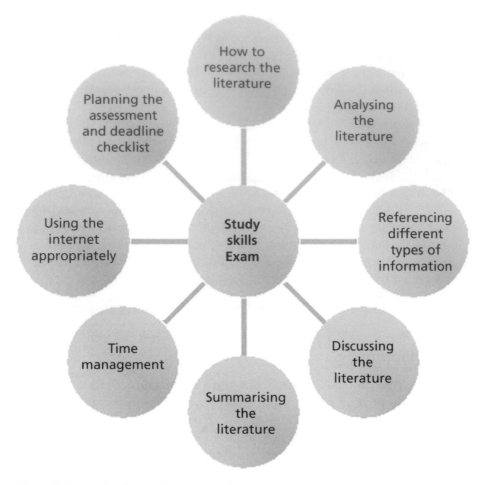

Figure 2 Example of a mind map or spider diagram

As you can see from the above basic diagram, finding information is not the only thing you have to think about when preparing for an assessment. However, finding the right information is more important than finding a large amount of useless information. When writing a report or exam your plan or mind map will help you to keep focused and prevent you becoming overwhelmed by the amount of information out there.

REFERENCING FROM JOURNALS AND BOOKS

Some students are never quite clear whether they should be using journals or books for their information requirements. More frequently, students will use the internet to search for information but this can lead them into more problems when referencing if they do not know how to do this properly. Chapter 1 has provided you with the basic support needed to search resources successfully and, more times than not, you will have found yourself looking at a book or a journal article either online or in your library. Websites are not usually very reliable as they can crash, be altered or be removed altogether. A student's preference for either books or journals becomes apparent when the submitted piece of work includes a reference list of only one or the other. This immediately informs the tutor that the student may be having problems when looking for information. As a basic rule, if your assignment is purely theoretical, books will usually be sufficient. However, if you are talking about practice, which you will be in health and social care, there also needs to be some evidence. Not many books simply provide evidence because their content is mainly the opinion of the author, whereas journal articles tend to provide the evidence in the form of research reports and analysis. A mixture of both books and journals in the references demonstrates an awareness of reliable information sources and the ability to apply them both. Chapter 2 explains how to reference the information that you have found but you should also remember that the way in which it is presented within your assignment is just as important. This will inform the reader whether you have understood the information and where you have looked for it. Referencing Wikipedia is therefore not good practice as it means that you have not looked very far or read any of the original work.

For some assignments you may be expected to have carried out a literature review. This usually means a search of available information on evidence-based practice and research. Lindsay (2007) suggests that evidence-based practice can mean anything from research to individual stories so it is important to be able to understand what it is you are reviewing. In particular he suggests that it is always worthwhile searching the 'grey literature', which means projects and studies that have not been published in books or journals but may be found in project reports and dissertations.

ORGANISING AND COMPOSING YOUR WORK

The next stage is to find and record information on the ideas you have identified in your plan. This is not something that is always taught in higher education and has been identified as a barrier for people who enter higher education after the age of 18, who are the first in the family to go to HE or who are from different cultural backgrounds. The information may be found from journals, books, the internet and/or the media, and this has been discussed in more detail in Chapters 1 and 2. However, you will also need to organise your detailed notes somewhere that you can access them easily. This may be in a simple notebook or an electronic source such as Refworks™ or Endnote™. Again, you will need to become familiar fairly quickly with these programmes so that they will be of use to you throughout the course. You may prefer to use an index box system with individual cards for references and notes from sources you have accessed. You will then begin to join all the information together just as you did in the mind map but, this time, it will be joined by paragraphs. It is important that your work makes sense to the reader, as this will inevitably make it easier to read and mark. For research reports you may want to follow a model of information gathering such as the PICO (Stone 2002) or SPICE (Beecroft *et al.*, 2006) models which are outlined below.

The PICO model

- Patient/problem
- Intervention
- Comparison
- Outcome

The SPICE model

- Setting
- Perspective
- Intervention
- Comparison
- Evaluation

Whatever method of organisation and composition you choose you will need to have your work finished in plenty of time for proofreading. This entails checking that your writing is grammatically correct and that there are no spelling errors in the work. You will have realised by now that managing your time is a very good way of staying organised and keeping to your plan. Time management is discussed in more detail in Chapter 8 and you may need to evaluate this skill from time to time to see if it needs improving. Some common signs of poor time management include:

- untidy presentation;
- late submissions;
- frequent extension requests;
- last-minute writing/tutorial requests;
- poor referencing;
- poor grammar;
- lack of proofreading (evident from frequent spelling mistakes).

You may be able to add more to this list but if you can you probably need to be looking at your own time management skills. There may be problems appearing that you identified at the planning stage but did nothing about, or there may have been unforeseen events over which you had no control. Whatever is interfering with your time management, you need to deal with it sooner rather than later. Falling behind with coursework will put extra pressure and strain upon your already precious time; dealing with problems promptly prevents small problems from becoming out of control. Poor time management can also contribute to a poor mark, which is disappointing to everyone, especially if you have worked so hard on the other aspects of writing your assignment. You may have spent too much time on aspects such as finding the evidence or planning, leaving you little time to write the assignment. If this is the case you will need to look again at your deadline checklist in your diary.

When composing your work you will need to look at what level of composition is expected from you. These should relate to the learning outcomes for each assignment. Academic levels are set by the Quality Assurance Agency and are different for each level of study (see Figure 3).

- Certificate – demonstrate knowledge of different concepts and ideas from the literature.
- Diploma – demonstrate knowledge and understanding (discussion) of different concepts.
- Degree – demonstrate awareness and critical analysis of evidence-based practice (research).
- Masters – able to critically evaluate research methodologies and apply to practice.
- Doctorate – ability to critically analyse and understand existing knowledge and create new knowledge.

Figure 3 Levels of higher education study (adapted from the QAA Framework, 2001)

As can be seen from Figure 3, the composition of your work needs to attain at least the level of your study and be able to demonstrate your ability to achieve that level. The levels are deliberately non-specific but each course tutor should be able to incorporate the level descriptors into the learning outcomes. This is why it is important to check your own work to see if you have achieved them.

Activity

Organising and composing your work

If you are not sure how your work should be laid out go back to a book or journal article that you have used for your assignment. You can develop your own critical analysis skills by asking the following questions.

- How have the author(s) organised their work?
- How have they referenced the information within the text?
- Do they present an argument within the text or is it just describing something?
- Is it the authors' own opinion or have they used research to support their claims?

ENGINEERING YOUR WORK AND WRITING REPORTS

You may also need to write your assignment in different formats depending upon what the assignment or examination brief requires, or if you are writing a literature review or a research report. It is important therefore to be aware of the different requirements. However, developing your own writing style is also important and once you have found what you are comfortable with you will be able to develop your own style more successfully throughout your course. Some students are sculptors who shape and change their work carefully as they go along, while others are engineers who build it up into a solid construction with little change (Lloyd, 2007). Your module tutor may also prefer a particular writing style so it would be wise to check with them to see, for example, if you are required to use headings or not, or if they have any other style preferences.

A written assignment should always include an introduction, to tell the reader where you are going with your analysis, and a conclusion to tell the reader where you have been. The introduction and conclusion are not the same, however, and each should justify their own existence by saying why you have chosen to focus upon a particular area and conclude with what you have learned during the process. This demonstrates that you have understood the brief and have done your best to answer it within the parameters of the word/time length of the assignment/exam.

Writing a report is slightly different from an assignment or exam in that, depending upon the type of report, you will be required to include certain headings. With a research report, for example, you are expected to include the following information.

- Title.
- Abstract.
- Introduction and background information.
- Literature review.
- Methods of data collection and analysis.
- Results.
- Discussion.
- Limitations.
- Conclusion.
- Acknowledgements.

This is a fairly standardised approach to writing reports that many tutors and examiners would expect to see within the assignment (Silverman, 2006). However, it is only likely that you will be required to complete this type of report when you are studying at degree level and above. For more information on writing this type of assignment see Chapter 6, which will help you organise your work further. However, your marks will reflect the spelling and structure of the assignment, whatever level you are studying at.

Activity

Obtaining feedback

Obtaining feedback and feed forward (Knight, 2007) is a very important part of the learning process but, unfortunately, it is not used to the best advantage. Spend a few minutes thinking about when you last obtained feedback on something that you did well or not so well and how it made you feel about your learning. Also think about any formative assessments you have undertaken (a tutorial can be included in this). Were you given feedback on how to improve your mark and, more importantly, did you use it?

SPELLING AND STRUCTURE

The course tutors usually provide marking guidelines so that students can see what their work will be marked against – this is different from the assignment brief. Some are very elaborate, with each section broken down into individual marks, while others are what are known as grade related, where the marker is free to mark within the grade. If you are provided with marking guidelines, please use them to assess your own standard of work. Some students are now being asked to assess some part of their work themselves and, by becoming their own critic, they can learn how to develop some of their weaker academic writing skills. However, marking guidelines are simply that – guidelines – and they cannot really demonstrate the complex decision making that takes place when lecturers assess your work. It is argued that lecturers should be more flexible in setting assessments to accommodate the different needs of students but, in reality, and mainly due to time constraints, the written word is still the main area of assessment. However, this should not be seen as a simple measurement of achievement, i.e. if I do this and that I will get an A, but a complex judgement of the whole piece of work that accumulates throughout the programme of study (Knight, 2007). Tutorials with your tutor are therefore very important if you want to achieve the best possible grade or mark, as they will be able to give you their professional advice and opinion on your work. This may include advice on explaining a term in more depth or making sure you have supported your work from the literature you have read. It is very easy to become so immersed in your work that you miss the point of demonstrating your understanding rather than expecting the reader to guess whether you truly understand a concept.

Writing in the first or third person

Students are often confused about whether they should write in the first or third person. When writing in the first person the work in general is usually accepted as being less formal. In this book we have written in the first person to generate a feeling of informality with you the student. This style of writing is often used in books or where a more personal relationship needs to be developed to get your message across. It does not depend upon the level of study; many doctoral students use the first person when talking about their research. However, if the work is a more formal piece then writing in the third person is more appropriate. This means that we do not write about me or you (first or second person) but about people, subjects, participants, authors (the third person) who are less familiar to us. It also demonstrates an ability to be objective within our writing, instead of subjective, and helps us move away from our own opinions towards theoretically informed discussion and analysis. There are arguments therefore for using either first or third person writing but a general rule is that if you are writing about your own experience use 'I' but, if not, use 'the author'.

CONCLUSION

Students who are embarking upon a period of study need to learn the process very quickly and this can be daunting, even for those whose family and/or friends have already been through the process. This chapter has outlined the assessment process of assignments, report writing and examinations in relation to the levels of study within a programme. However, you will need to develop individual skills in planning, gathering and organising information, and managing your own time alongside this process. With some careful preparation and support from the people in place to help, you should quickly become familiar with this new language and feel comfortable in discussing your own needs with tutors and peers.

Summary

- A plan is the best way to begin your writing and guide your study time.

- Using your referenced material wisely demonstrates good understanding.

- Organising and composing your work correctly will help you meet that deadline.

- Engineering your writing style will develop your academic writing skills.

- The spelling and structure of your work gives an overall impression of your ability.

5

Learning in Groups and Teams

Liz Lefroy

Learning outcomes

In this chapter you will learn how to:

- apply theories about how groups and teams work;

- develop some of the skills required for successful group/team functioning;

- identify the values that underpin group/team learning activities.

INTRODUCTION

Many students enter higher education with both a personal ambition to gain a qualification and a wish to learn with others. Those studying for health and social care qualifications will also be aware that they will be required to work in teams on placement. Just as an ability to learn alone is essential in higher education, so learning with others in the classroom or on placement is a key skill. Group learning can bring benefits and opportunities not available to the lone student. Cottrell (1999) identifies some of these: students can share ideas, gain extra perspectives and stimulate each other's thinking. Skills such as these will benefit the student beyond the point of qualification. The National Occupational Standards for Social Workers, for example, state that social workers must 'Contribute to evaluating the effectiveness of the team, network or system' (TOPSS, 2002, Key Role 5, 17.3). Therefore, for students in health and social care, learning in groups and teams has a dual purpose. It enhances the learning experience, but it will also prepare students for professional practice. This chapter focuses on aspects of the knowledge, skills and values students need to get the best out of group learning situations, whether these are encountered in the classroom or on placement.

Some definitions

Service users, carers and patients

Labelling people, particularly those from groups that are marginalised, is problematic. Descriptive vocabulary is necessary, however, so the most commonly accepted terms – service users and carers (in relation to social care services) and patients (in relation to health services) – are used in this chapter.

Groups and teams

There are differences of opinion about the definition of groups and teams. Much of the literature concerning teamwork is written from a business perspective and, in this context, teams are prized over groups. However, within social care and health, the distinction is not as clear, nor is the term 'group' perceived as negative. In the context of this chapter, the groups and teams described are likely to share many characteristics and to be equal in value and complexity.

KNOWLEDGE AND THEORY

Scenario 1

Jo is in her first year of a social work degree. She had been looking forward to meeting her classmates and the first week together went well. She was upset by the end of the second week, however, as some members of the class seemed more interested in competing with other students than in learning. Others seemed content to 'sit back' while their colleagues did the work. Jo also could not understand why she found Patrick's contributions to discussions so irritating. While Jo is keen to reach conclusions, Patrick seems to focus on the details of the discussions.

Theories can be useful as 'maps' for understanding human situations and interactions, sometimes providing distance between an incident and an emotional response. If students can formulate ideas about why a particular group learning experience is difficult, for example, they will be less likely to blame themselves, each other or their tutors and to work towards a constructive resolution. The experience of student Jo, above, can be better understood if the following theories are taken into consideration.

Group learning theories

There are many theories about how students learn (see Chapter 3 on Learning Styles for further examples). In terms of group learning, however, the work of Sylvia Downs is a useful illustration. According to Downs (1993) learning is composed of three components: facts, concepts and physical skills, which, in turn, involve processes of memorising, understanding and doing (MUD). While memorising is a task perhaps suited to solo learning, Downs found that, if understanding is required, students working in groups tend to learn more than those working alone. By recognising the different aspects or dimensions of learning, as revealed through learning theories, it becomes clearer which types of learning may best be achieved in groups or teams.

In addition to the MUD taxonomy of learning, Downs identified that many adult learners have developed learning blockages that make effective learning difficult. Downs found (1993) that the most common areas of difficulty are:

- poor learning skills;
- poor concentration;
- worries/fears about learning;
- difficulty in learning from others.

Learning in groups may help adults to overcome blockages such as poor concentration and deficiencies in learning skills. It is clear, however, that other blockages, such as anxiety and difficulty in learning from others, will be compounded in group learning situations. Blockages may be demonstrated in behaviour such as the 'social loafing' described by Alpay (2005, p.10). This is a situation in which a group member expects to be carried by others' efforts. A student may be only too happy, for reasons of lack of confidence, motivation or skills, to remain quiet within a group, to use the ideas/skills of others but to contribute little.

The 'Life-Cycle' of groups and teams

A useful theory when considering groups and teams is that of Tuckman (1965) who described groups as going through a process of 'forming, storming, norming and performing'. The forming stage is the process of people getting together. In Scenario 1, Jo's experience was that this was an exciting and positive time. Later on, however, the group seemed to undergo a 'storming' phase: a struggle between students to establish their positions within the group. The likelihood is that if the class follows Tuckman's model, a stage of 'norming' will evolve in which the students will recognise the need to work together. Once they have achieved this, the class can get on with 'performing', focusing on its purpose.

Learning from Practice 1

How does this service user's account of her membership of a committee relate to Tuckman's theory?

I was asked to join a newly commissioned service as a committee member and independent service user. The service had been awarded the contract to provide advocacy for users of secondary mental health services. Its remit was to be service user led. I had been involved in the commissioning process so I had existing knowledge about what was required and the needs of service users in the area. It is a very positively driven committee because the service is much needed by everyone.

At first it was difficult because all the other committee members knew each other (they had worked together previously). It took me some time to learn about the people, the organisations involved, the terminology they used and how the service could be developed. Having two other service users on the committee, as well as people whose expertise was in this area meant I could access the support and information I needed more easily. However, it took time for me to feel at ease doing this.

Fifteen months on, I feel I am an equal member of the committee. My views are sought, listened to and respected and I have now been asked to chair the committee. I now feel comfortable both about influencing decisions and acknowledging when I do not understand issues. I think this comes with time and feeling secure within that group of people.

Team Role Theory

Another theory, which will help the student to understand the anatomy of teams, is the highly influential Team Role Theory of Meredith Belbin.

Belbin found that there are nine roles that can be represented in a team. These roles can be shared or an individual can fulfil two or three of the roles. Belbin (1981) identified the following roles:

- **Shaper** – this person is driven and wants to make progress towards goals quickly. She keeps a team focused and active. In Scenario 1, Jo could be described as a shaper.

- **Plant** – this person is creative and has many ideas, which are not necessarily practical but can be turned into reality by the team.

- **Monitor Evaluator** – this person questions what the group is doing. This can seem as if he is undermining the work of the group. In fact his questioning can prevent the team from making mistakes.

- **Completer Finisher** – this person has an eye for detail, spotting gaps and errors. The Shaper and the Completer Finisher may irritate each other, just as Jo and Patrick do in Scenario 1.

- **Implementer** – this person can take a problem and work out how to solve it. Her practical approach may sometimes clash with the Plant's innovative ideas.

- **Resource Investigator** – this person can help the team to solve its problems by networking outside the team.

- **Team Worker** – this person helps to facilitate the interpersonal relationships within the team.

- **Co-ordinator** – this person ensures that all members of the team have their say. He understands that listening to all views can result in better decisions.

- **Specialist** – this person brings specialist knowledge to the team. The service user's or patient's role in a group may include that of specialist.

Activity

Understanding the theory of group/team functioning
Jo (Scenario 1) could use theory to understand what is happening in her class. Can theory help you to understand any group situations, positive or negative, that you are currently experiencing?

SKILLS

Scenario 2

Carlton, a social work student, was pleased to gain a first year placement in a Children and Families team as he had previously worked as a support worker in a children's home. He was sure he could contribute as well as learning from the experience.

In his first team meeting, he joined in a discussion of a service user's case on the spur of the moment. He was nervous and unable to express himself clearly and spoke in a flat tone of voice. Lisa was fidgeting as Carlton spoke and cut across him with a different viewpoint, referring as she did so to Carlton's view as 'green'.

Carlton approached his placement tutor after the meeting for advice about dealing with the situation, which had undermined his already fragile confidence.

The complex nature of interpersonal relationships, in addition to the different perspectives of team roles, makes conflict a frequent experience in group learning. Groups and teams in which communication is poor can at best not fulfil their potential and at worst operate in an atmosphere of conflict. Students, while they may often feel relatively powerless, can nevertheless learn skills that will ensure a better outcome in group or team situations not only for themselves but also for other participants

Communication

The most important skills needed within groups and teams are communication skills. 'Communication' states Thompson (2003, p. 1), 'is not a simple mechanical matter of passing information from one person to one or more others but rather is a complex multilevel event.' The Department for Education and Skills (DfES, 2005, p. 6) describes communication as follows:

Good communication is central to working with children, young people, their families and carers . . . It involves listening, questioning, understanding and responding to what is being communicated by children, young people and those caring for them . . . Communication is not just about the words you use, but also your manner of speaking, body language and, above all, the effectiveness with which you listen.

Learning in groups crucially involves listening to others. Listening involves not only giving others a chance to speak but also a positive demonstration that what has been said has been heard (Cottrell, 1999). This is called active listening and incorporates skills such as nodding to show understanding, giving eye contact, smiling and avoiding distracting others by fidgeting. These skills need to reflect individual needs so, for example, a person with a visual impairment would need audible rather than visual feedback.

Paralanguage concerns the way in which something is said, rather than what is said. In Scenario 2, Lisa may have been distracted from what Carlton was saying by his flat tone of voice and other signs of nervousness. The work of Albert Mehrabian is often cited in relation to non-verbal communication. In experiments conducted in the 1960s he famously found that communication is 7 per cent verbal (the actual words you use), 38 per cent vocal (tone of voice, inflection) and 55 per cent non-verbal (appearance, body language) (Mehrabian, 1972). This work has been criticised as being of limited applicability, even by Mehrabian himself: clearly the distribution of meaning will be different for different people in different situations. However, it demonstrates something important. Saying one thing but communicating something else through tone or body language is called 'incongruence'. Learning in groups gives students the opportunities to learn and practise skills of congruence.

Learning from Practice 2

Here is an account from a service user about the impact of paralanguage.

I needed to challenge a professional on a personal comment made to me in a training session in which I was one of the trainers. Our views on the context of the comment differed hugely.

The professional related their account, but my perspective differed and I was deeply shocked as I thought what the professional said was untrue. As I spoke, asked questions and tried to reason with the professional, she was unable to make eye contact and was often unable to talk directly to me, and was constantly moving position.

This disagreement could not be resolved, but because of this body language, I felt that my challenge had been justified. It made me very aware of the wariness some service users feel when trying to talk about their needs to staff.

While the service user's experiences emphasise the point that communication is not just about words, the words you use are important. Words can be used to discriminate or oppress. An example of this is the way that professionals can use jargon that prevents service users and patients from understanding. Furthermore, words can convey unintended meanings. Students need to develop what Thompson (2003) describes as linguistic sensitivity. The word 'handicapped' has, for example, been rejected by disabled people as pejorative, incorporating as it does the notion of dependence and charity (cap in hand). Such sensitivity is often dismissed as mere political correctness, but this attitude denies the reality that language can reinforce unequal power relationships.

Learning focus

In developing linguistic sensitivity, avoid words that exclude – for example, use 'firefighter' not 'fireman'. Avoid language that depersonalises – for example, use 'elderly people' or 'older people' rather than 'the elderly'. Avoid language that stigmatises – for example, use of the word 'mental' in a derogatory way. Avoid stereotypes – for example, jokes that rely on a notion of Irish people as stupid.

Emotional intelligence

Students rarely have the choice to opt out of a group in which they feel uncomfortable. Instead, they need to learn the skills to change how they feel. Goleman (1996) describes the core aspects of emotional intelligence as managing one's own and others' emotions. These fundamental skills, which have traditionally been overlooked in an eagerness to measure IQ (intelligence quotient), are crucial to the successful functioning of groups.

Goleman identifies the ability of a group to harmonise as the group's emotional quotient (EQ). A high EQ leads to the most productive and creative groups and teams:

> The single most important factor in maximizing the excellence of a group's product was the degree to which the members were able to create a state of internal harmony, which lets them take advantage of the full talents of their members.
>
> (Goleman, 1996, p. 161)

In Scenario 2 Carlton's potentially valuable contribution is being dismissed. Carlton's nervous communication seems to have reinforced a prejudice Lisa holds about the value of student contribution to the team. While responsibility lies with Lisa for her prejudice, Carlton is not as powerless as he may feel. He can choose to manage Lisa's response to him by taking some positive steps. By acknowledging his own feelings of anxiety and by trying to understand what Lisa is feeling about having a new student in the team, Carlton can, with his placement tutor's help, take steps towards a more constructive outcome at the next team meeting. Carlton's placement tutor may, for example, advise him to prepare in advance for team meetings as a way of building confidence. Carlton could request an agenda and develop some written points. Instead of his paralanguage conveying nervousness, referring to notes would make it clear that he had prepared for the meeting. Carlton could practise making points slowly, ensuring he conveys enthusiasm in a lively tone of voice. After the meeting, a short period of reflection on what went well, what could have gone better and what would be good to change for next time (perhaps written up as a reflective account for his placement portfolio) would help Carlton to focus on what was positive about the experience. This process of preparation, action and reflection will enable Carlton to manage his emotions within the team.

Students need to be able to control their emotional responses in group and team situations and to be able to empathise with others. Actively considering others' feelings, being aware that they too may feel anxious, for example, is a first step towards empathy. Together with self-management, empathy is the emotional skill needed in what Goleman describes as 'the art of handling relationships' (1996, p. 112). A group can raise its EQ by, for example, acknowledging at the start of a session that people have come to it from a variety of situations and with a variety of emotions. Another example is to agree as a group the rules for giving and receiving constructive criticism (see below).

Managing conflicts

Thompson (2000, p. 60) states, 'one of the difficulties of understanding interactions is that we are usually part of the dynamic that we are trying to understand . . .' Learning in groups and teams can be immensely rewarding, but it can also result in conflict. A sound knowledge and values base and good communication skills will diminish the likelihood of serious conflict. Nevertheless, conflicts can result from differences of opinion and, crucially, the way in which individuals interact or express those disagreements.

Conflict can arise when people feel criticised. By definition, students' work will be evaluated during their degree and they may also be required to give feedback to others. The ability to give and receive constructive criticism can minimise opportunities for conflict and is a useful skill underpinned by an attitude that regards criticism, or feedback, as an opportunity for learning.

Lisa (Scenario 2) could learn from Cottrell (1999, p. 99) who describes some techniques for offering constructive criticism, including:

- agreeing first within the group about whether criticism will be offered;
- offering praise for what is good;
- looking to future potential changes, rather than going over what has already happened;
- avoiding commenting on people (for example, say 'That statement might be seen as discriminatory' rather than 'You are so prejudiced!');
- not criticising everything – choosing one or two points to make;
- using a warm tone of voice and open body language that will convey support rather than hostility.

A list such as this can form the basis for discussion within a group or team about how feedback will be given. Ground rules such as these can, simply by being discussed in advance, change group behaviour.

Carlton needs advice from his practice learning tutor about how to deal with Lisa's behaviour if it is repeated in future. The following student activity gives insight into what his best response might be.

Activity

Managing conflict in groups

In a team meeting a case you have been working on is being discussed. You are taken by surprise when your placement tutor criticises some work that you have done. While you think she may have some useful feedback for you, she has not previously mentioned this and you feel the way she has raised this issue is unfair. What do you do?

1. Nothing – challenging her would be too risky as she has the power to pass or fail your placement.

2. Thank her for her feedback, making it clear that you have not heard this opinion before. Explain the reasons why you took the particular actions being discussed and suggest you would value the team's comments.

3. Confront her, saying, 'It's not fair that you have raised this issue without discussing it with me first.'

4. Telephone your college tutor after the meeting to complain about the placement tutor's actions.

5. Speak to the placement tutor after the meeting, explaining why her approach seemed unfair to you.

The best answer here is 2. You have controlled your emotional responses but you are also rejecting the placement tutor's abuse of power and insensitivity in this situation. A confrontation would not be as effective in making your point and would reflect badly on you. The option to speak to her or to your college tutor in private may seem appealing, but would still leave you with the feeling that you had not stood up for yourself when treated badly.

VALUES

Scenario 3

This extract, written by a service user, demonstrates some of the values necessary for successful team and group working.

Five years ago I was asked to be involved in suicide awareness and risk training for mental health service staff. There was no precedent for this work so there was no previous service user experience to draw on.

My contribution started as an account of my personal experience – a 'living case study'. It evolved into training that I was fully involved in designing, delivering, evaluating and developing – in fact it ended up at a totally different point from where it started!

There was a lot of learning and give and take on all sides throughout the process and I felt much happier delivering the training than I had with my original talk.

As a service user, having my experience and expertise valued and used in this way allowed me to use skills I developed in my professional life and I found this very empowering. I think this was an example of a gold standard of service user/patient involvement. I truly became a member of the team and this should always be the aim.

Whenever students communicate with each other, with tutors, service users, patients, carers and professionals they communicate something of the relationship concerned. This can be, for example, one of co-operation and equality, or one of authoritarian oppression (Thompson, 2003). Teams and groups that are based upon values of mutual respect and a celebration of diversity can achieve the 'gold standard' of partnership described in Scenario 3. Learning in groups and teams provides students with opportunities to reflect upon and develop the values necessary to achieve such partnership.

Respect and partnership

The principle value of any social care or health student must be one of respect for people based on a belief that respect is a universal right, rather than on any notion of respect having to be earned. This perspective provides a basis for relationships with service users and patients, colleagues and fellow students. Students may argue that this principle can be taken as a given, but examples of poor practice cited by patients and service users, such as that in Learning from Practice 2, demonstrate that this cannot be taken for granted.

One reason for this is that understanding of what constitutes respect can vary between individuals, cultures, professions and organisations. As a result, professional bodies, in consultation with service users and patients, describe what respect means in the professional context. An example of this is the Code of Practice for social care workers (General Social Care Council 2002), which lists, among other attributes, honesty (2.1), reliability (2.4, 2.5) and confidentiality (2.3) as behavioural requirements.

Definitions of respect are further broadened by the academic standards, such as those set out by the Department of Health in the social work subject benchmark statements. These specify a requirement to:

> Involve users of social work services in ways that increase their resources, capacity and power to influence factors affecting their lives [and to] consult actively with others, including service users, who hold relevant information or expertise.
>
> (DoH, 2002, 3.2.4)

Social workers are required to work (both at the level of the provision of care and support to the individual and at the wider level of service planning and development) in a way which actively values the views and expertise of service users, patients and carers (Warren, 2007).

These levels of partnership are not limited to the social worker–service user relationship in practice, but are increasingly being extended into higher education. The participation of service users and carers has been made central to the degree in social work. For example, the Care Council for Wales' *Standards on Involving Service Users and Carers in Social Work Education* (2005) states that, 'service users and carers are involved in developing and delivering teaching and learning opportunities in colleges and agencies as contributors with equally valued expertise' (Standard 8, p. 23).

Students need to understand that approaches in higher education are evolving. The model of learning now is, at its best, one of partnership: of a team in which student, service user, lecturer and placement tutor collaborate to achieve the best outcome.

Diversity as strength

Respect for individuals must be coupled with recognition of diversity as strength for such teams to fulfil their learning potential. Thus, it is not simply a matter of tolerating, accommodating or recognising that different opinions, cultures and experiences exist. Understanding that diversity enriches learning and the planning and delivery of services is essential. Diversity 'implies not just gender and race, age and disability but also difference in experience, in functional competence, in attitudes and culture' (Singh, 2002, p. 23). Singh goes on to cite the research of Maznesvski (1994) demonstrating that diverse teams 'lead to the emergence of new and valuable viewpoints, enabling better quality decision-making' (p. 23). These findings are reinforced by the service user's experience in Scenario 3 in which the outcome was unexpected, and better, because of service user involvement.

Viewing diversity in the terms Singh describes may challenge perceptions of service users and patients. Students may have joined courses in social care or health with vague notions of wanting to 'help people'. Recognising diversity as strength shifts the view away from seeing service users and patients as needy and dependent and 'offers alternative models upon which to base our relationships with them' (Warren, 2007, p. 4). Moreover, groups of students studying for the same degree are likely to have some similarities in terms of experience and educational attainment. It is the differences in experience and viewpoints within the student group, however, which will provide the most opportunities for learning.

Activity

Behaviour to avoid in group/team learning
Having considered constructive ways to improve the quality of experience of learning in groups and teams, identify five behaviours to avoid in future group/team scenarios.

Summary

In this chapter, we have considered some key areas of knowledge and skills needed for successful learning in groups and teams. These have included aspects of:

- group learning theory;
- group life-cycles;
- team role theory;
- communication;
- emotional intelligence;
- conflict management.

- The underpinning values of respect, partnership and recognising diversity as strength have also been highlighted as essential for teams and groups to achieve effectiveness.
- Students must, in addition, recognise their own responsibility in ensuring that the groups and teams of which they are a part become the best possible learning environments not only for themselves, but also for fellow students, professionals, patients and service users with whom they work and learn.

The author gratefully acknowledges the contributions of Anne Dennis, service user, to this chapter.

6

Effective and Efficient Reading Skills and Note Taking

Marjorie Lloyd

Learning outcomes

At the end of this chapter you will be able to:

- find appropriate information quickly and efficiently;
- write clear and concise notes;
- be able to plan a review of the literature.

FINDING THE RIGHT INFORMATION

This chapter will help you to develop your understanding of the different types of information available and will build upon the skills you have developed in previous chapters. One problem that students in higher education often have is the feeling of being overwhelmed by the amount of information that is available to them and they often wonder where they should actually start looking. To begin with, and before you can start looking for information for your assignment, you should spend some time thinking about what type of information you will need. This will differ for the different assignments that you are given so do not be afraid initially to cast your net as wide as possible to help you explore the vast amount of information available. Only then can you begin to narrow it down to the most appropriate information that you will need.

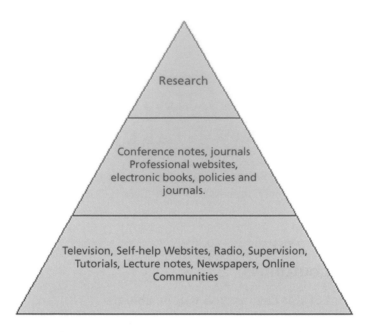

Figure 1 Types of information available

Figure 1 provides an overview of the many forms of information that you may be thinking about but, for academic purposes, you will also need to be thinking about which types of information will provide you with the most accurate evidence for your assignment. The Quality Assurance Agency (2006c) (see the introduction to this book for more information) requires higher education establishments to demonstrate that you have achieved a level of learning by providing evidence for that level of learning (see Chapter 4 for more information on levels of learning). Therefore, you will be expected to have explored beyond the everyday information that is available to all of society, such as that found in newspapers and websites, to other more challenging arguments for your ideas. While it may be useful to use quotations from the media to provide examples of what you will be studying you will also need to explain why you have used a quotation and how this may influence your writing.

Activity

Finding appropriate information
Read the following and consider whether it would be suitable for an assignment. You may want to make a note of why you think it is suitable or not, for discussion with your tutor.

My brother's first joint and his descent into a mental war zone

The *Observer*, Sunday 13 January 2008, Alexander Linklater

In the summer of 2005, there was nothing particularly new about the onset of one of my brother's episodes. It was frustrating and sad, because Archie had at that point been doing well for some time and there is always the faint hope in manic depression that a remission might somehow take root and become permanent. But the symptoms were familiar enough: restlessness, the sudden announcement of grandiose plans, bouts of rage – and then the wild paroxysms of mood and personality that can lead to psychosis. Or madness, as Archie prefers to call it.

What was slightly different was the recent appearance of news reports on further studies into the links between cannabis and mental illness, with the emphasis on a genetic vulnerability to the drug. It was a subject that had gradually been worming its way into public consciousness, and my family felt the potential implications acutely.

The above exercise may help you to begin to plan how you will access information by following a certain lead or story and developing your assignment around it. There may also be other cues such as the assignment title – is it specific enough to tell you exactly where to start looking or is it so vague it could mean anything? Your tutor will help you get started if you are having difficulties but it is worth demonstrating that you have thought about the subject in advance of arranging a tutorial. You may also want to try out your mind mapping skills, which were discussed in Chapter 4.

Search engines

Electronic search engines are probably one of the most commonly used methods that today's students will use to find information quickly. Unfortunately, some of these search engines are more accurate than others and, if you do not define your search words adequately, you will discover thousands of links to your search. In addition, the information provided may not be of the standard required for you to develop your knowledge beyond common knowledge. Chapter 1 will help you to search for information more effectively using the internet. For example, Google™ is a very popular search engine and there are many other less well-known sites but you must remember that they are only search engines and they will find whatever you ask them to find. They will not determine whether what they find for you is reliable evidence – you will have to do that. Google™ does provide a 'Scholar' site, which will tell you in the search whether it is a book, a paper or a citation elsewhere and the link will direct you to the source. However, unless you have online subscriptions to the many journals available, or an unlimited book budget, you will soon find your search resulting in a dead end. It is therefore important and very useful to you to become familiar with the online journals and library catalogue within your university so that you will immediately know you are searching reputable and available sources. You may also use the library facility to put a hold on books (from home) and access online study guides provided by your university. Wherever possible it is better to use your own university guides rather than those provided by another university. While you may prefer the layout belonging to another university, your own university guidelines will be based upon the assessment criteria that will be used to mark your work. Most universities will subscribe to online journal search engines and will subscribe to some or all of the journals in the search engine. Therefore, you will know that whatever you do find you will be able to access the whole article/book and not be prevented by a subscription fee or denied access altogether.

Activity

Using search engines

You have already been introduced to using the internet to find information in Chapter 1. Now is the time to hone these new skills on finding information that you need quickly. You can practise this by typing in some key words into one of your university's search engines and test yourself on the following points:

1. How did you refine your search from too many to a manageable amount of links?
2. How long did it take you to get one document/book?
3. Did you change anything to speed up the process and, if so, what did you do?

These will be useful discussion points for tutorial or peer support.

Finding information quickly

When you have discovered an article or book that you think may be useful to you, you will need to find out if it is worth locating, printing or downloading the whole article or part of the book (there are copyright laws that do not allow you to copy more than a certain amount of text from a book). You will therefore need to scan the overall document to see if it is what you are looking for. You can do this by reading abstracts and looking at the subheadings. Alternatively, you will find that you can learn a great deal about what is in the book or article from the index and reference list and by looking for your keyword(s). Don't be convinced just by the title as these are often used to grab your attention and there are some interesting titles that have little or no relevance to what is actually in the paper. When you think that you have found what you are looking for you will have to speed-read or read very fast and yet still obtain the information that you need to support your assignment. The three Ss below may help you to remember that in order to find information quickly you will need to:

- **Scan** the document or book to
- **See** if it is actually what you are looking for and, if so, then
- **Speed-read** the whole document to find the information you are looking for.

Speed-reading is an activity that students will develop in an ad hoc way but it can be organised to save the student a great deal of time. There are also free computer packages such as Readpal™ available on the internet that will help you to skim through documents and some books on your computer screen. In an accompanying book, Crowe (2005) provides some useful advice on how to prepare yourself to read through a large amount of material in a short time. Some of the hints and tips provided in Crowe's book *Speed Reading* are:

- clear your desk space of anything that you will not be reading/using;
- make sure you have a quiet space and time slot in order to read with no distractions;
- playing music can help to relax you and block out background noise but music with lyrics will distract you;
- make sure you have some way of making notes to make best use of the time or you will forget what you have read;
- take regular breaks to aid concentration, move around every 30 minutes or so and take a complete break every couple of hours.

In addition, it may be useful to vary the methods you use for gathering information, as reading can be difficult if you are tired from a hard day at work or studying. Podcasts are downloadable audio articles that often provide information from the literature and latest research or you can listen to discussion broadcasts such as those from BBC Radio 4, for example. Alternatively, why not look for some web casts or video casts of news items and speeches. Some well-known authors (and lecturers) are also becoming more familiar with web logs, which are online journals or diaries used to record their current thinking, that would be useful in supporting your information. Try looking at the web logs from your university if these are available, or those on current health and social care journal websites such as the *Community Care* journal website. Finally, online (social networking) communities such as Facebook™, Beebo™ and MySpace™, etc. are becoming a growing networking and group learning area with some students finding their layout and informality a preferable place to the formal environment of the non-virtual classroom. The problem with this development in learning and finding information is that whereas students have developed this informal networking skill quickly with the easy availability of technology today, some tutors have not quite caught up. This means that there is currently a difference of opinion about what represents valid 'evidence' for your work and this will be an issue that each university will be addressing separately. There is no doubt that e-learning will become a more frequent mode of learning and gathering information but you should expect it to be a bumpy journey for the next few years. Lindsay (2007, p. xi) suggests that evidence-based practice means:

> using the best evidence you have about the most effective care of individuals, using it with the person's best interests in mind, to the best of your ability, and in such a way that it is clear that you are doing it.

MAKING CONCISE NOTES

When students first begin higher education study they seem to need to write down every word that is said by a lecturer or every word that describes some concept in a book or journal. Students soon learn that, with the amount of studying required, this becomes impossible and they need to find a way of making more concise notes. This is a skill that is usually developed on an individual basis but there are some useful approaches that will help you save time later.

- Always record the full reference so that you do not have to go looking for it later.
- Record words that are not familiar to you as a reminder to go and find out what they mean.
- If you are using quotations then always record the page number of the quote.
- Try and write information in your own words as this can help you to avoid plagiarism (remember that you will still need to reference the idea as belonging to someone else).
- Keep a notebook and pen with you at all times – an A5 size notebook is not too big or too small to carry around.
- Loose-leaf notepads are not ideal as pages can become detached and lost.

A good habit to acquire is that of making an annotated bibliography as you read your books or journals. An annotated bibliography helps you record concisely the main ideas within a text and, if it is written well, it can simply be transferred into your assignment with a linking sentence.

Example

An annotated bibliography entry

Kitwood (1997) argues that people who suffer from dementia are neglected in that professionals only focus upon their medical needs rather than the whole person. Kitwood suggests that there are many ways of helping people with dementia and that they should be acknowledged as people with a disability that has social consequences as much as, if not more than, medical consequences. He suggests that staff should attempt to develop relationships with people who suffer from dementia in order to maintain their 'personhood', and warns that a lack of therapeutic relationships may result in social 'malignancy'.

Kitwood, T. (1997) *Dementia Reconsidered: the person comes first.* Buckingham: Open University Press

---

Your annotated bibliography enables you to read the literature in more detail but, instead of taking copious notes, you will be taking from your reading what you think are the main points. This will save you time later when you start putting the assignment together as it will be a simple task of cutting and pasting your text into the assignment. This is also a useful skill to start working on for later in your programme when you may need to write a literature review. This can be an assignment on its own or a chapter within a larger assignment or dissertation.

Activity

Writing an annotated bibliography
Find a recent article or book that you have read and practise writing an annotated bibliography entry for it. Try to remember that this is not just a writing exercise but a useful skill that, when used with confidence, can save you time. Remember the following points when writing your bibliography entry:

- keep your word limit to around 100 words;
- identify the main points, findings and/or arguments;
- record the whole reference and page numbers if using quotations.

WRITING A LITERATURE REVIEW

As your programme of study develops, you are more likely to be asked to write a literature review. This will most often occur in the third year of a degree programme but may also be begun in the second year or final year of a diploma or foundation degree. As frightening as it may seem, a literature review is simply a collection of articles or books that contribute towards a body of evidence. In the main, this will consist of current research and policy documentation that will require some critical analysis (see Chapter 10).

Scenario

Sally was coming to the end of her second year of a foundation degree on childcare and had been asked to write a 3 000-word literature review on poverty and childhood. Sally had never done this before and was not sure how to go about the task. She did not know what type of information she needed to look for or how to find it. From what you have read so far, what could you say to Sally to help her get started?

There are a number of issues to start thinking about when asked to review the literature on a current subject. The following list is a guide but, as your skills and confidence grow, you may want to add some more that are specific to your own needs. As well as developing your organisational and time management skills a literature review also demands the ability to find information quickly (see Chapter 1) and apply critical thinking skills to what you have found (see Chapter 10).

Issues to consider when planning to carry out a literature review

- **Plan** – in order to find information for a literature review, as Sally has been requested to do, she must first make a plan or mind map (see Chapter 4, page 57).
- **Keywords** – from her plan Sally will be able to pick out keywords that she will use to find more information.
- **Search** – to find more information on a subject Sally will use a hand search through individual journals or books and/or use a search engine.
- **Note taking** – Sally will need to make some record of what she has found, either as handwritten notes, as notes in a citation manager programme such as Refworks™ or Endnote™, or on a portable electronic device such as a laptop or hand-held computer.

In the above scenario, Sally might search using keywords such as 'poverty', 'children' and, perhaps, words relating to other areas that she may have read around such as 'social class', 'education', 'health', 'parenting' and 'income'. The more words used in a search engine the wider the search will be. However, a search can also be made using a smaller combination of the same words, for example 'child', 'health' and 'income'. As you practise using keywords to search the literature, you will become more familiar with what works best and in what combination, but be warned: this activity does take time and patience. Often when students say that they cannot find anything they have either searched too widely or too narrowly and have to learn that searching the literature is a study skill.

As you begin to gather information and, invariably, documentation you will need to consider how you will file the information so that you can find it quickly later. A simple filing box may be all that is needed but it is also worth getting into the habit of creating your annotated bibliographies. Alternatively you can do all this online using citation manager programmes such as Endnote™ or Refworks™.

Finding the evidence

Evidence-based practice as mentioned earlier is about applying what you have read to your practice and, as a student, you also need to be able to write about it. This requires some of the skills mentioned above, together with skills discussed in other chapters (see Chapters 4 and 10). Before you begin your own literature review, you may also want to explore in more detail the process of finding information to conduct a literature review as this will help you become more familiar with what is required.

Activity

Find a journal article from a professional journal in your area of practice. Without reading the content in too much detail scan the whole document for headings. You will quickly be able to recognise an original research article if it has the following headings within it (these are also discussed in Chapter 4 on writing a research report). If it does not have them then it is probably a theoretical or opinion article.

- Title.
- Abstract.
- Introduction and background information.
- Literature review.
- Methods of data collection and analysis.
- Results.
- Discussion.
- Limitations.
- Conclusion.
- Acknowledgements.

However, Lindsay (2007, p. 14) adds to this list. He suggests that the following critical questions may be useful in analysing the literature that you have found as they will help you to become more analytical of the research itself.

- How much research is already out there?
- Where does it come from?
- Who has produced it?
- Who paid for it?

- What methods have been used to produce it?
- How old is it?

Critical analysis skills are discussed in more detail in Chapter 10 but it is worthwhile remembering that even though you may have no intention of carrying out any research in the near future you will still need to know what information informs your practice and how reliable it is. As Lindsay (2007) suggests, while research may not be the only form of evidence it is – or should be – what is most widely used in policy documents both locally and nationally. Social policy is increasingly informing our practice in the form of guidance and law but it is the practitioners who will need to be able to analyse and convert policy into practice. Reading and writing skills are therefore an essential part of the practitioners' study skills toolkit in order to capture the right information at the right time.

CONCLUSION

Preparing to write your first assignment often fills the student with dread at the thought of getting it wrong or not being able to find any information. With some careful preparation from the beginning, you can quickly learn to develop you own learning style and skills that will enable you to produce work that will achieve good marks. It is important to remember to use all the resources available to you, including your tutor, as they are there to help, not hinder you, and you will also develop your own confidence in your academic ability. Learning good writing skills at this stage in your development will enable you to go on to write for publication when you feel more confident. Unfortunately, many postgraduates are unable to do this because they have not developed the skills or the confidence to do so (Canter and Fairbairn, 2006)

REVISION QUIZ

1. Which of the following can you use in an assignment?

- Newspaper articles.
- Websites.
- Television programmes.
- Lecture notes.
- Books.
- Journals.
- Radio programmes.
- Tutorials.
- Supervision notes.

- Research.
- Conference notes.
- Professional forums.

2. Name three online resources for sourcing different types of information.

3. Which of the following will you need when reading articles and/or books?

   - Enough space.
   - Pens and paper.
   - Enough time.
   - Playing songs by your favourite singer.
   - Making notes as you read.

4. Why should you learn how to take notes?

   - To save time.
   - To copy other people's work.
   - To make sure you have referenced properly.
   - To develop your study skills.

5. Writing an annotated bibliography helps you to (tick the answer you think is correct):

   - make copious notes;
   - record the main ideas within a text;
   - create a long reference list.

6. In order to carry out a literature review you will need to (tick the answer/answers you think is/are correct):

   - make a plan;
   - identify some keywords;
   - develop a way of storing the information found;
   - know everything about the subject.

7

Presentations and Public Speaking

Paul Jeorrett

Learning outcomes

In this chapter you will learn how to:

- identify keys to effective preparation, planning and practice for presentations in a range of circumstances;

- approach a presentation methodically;

- identify good and poor practice when delivering presentations;

- effectively use presentation software and other media to enhance a presentation.

INTRODUCTION

Presentations and public speaking are critical in nearly all professional careers in the twenty-first century. Presentation skills are vital in communicating information, presenting and promoting youself and your ideas and in sharing knowledge with groups of all sizes and in many contexts, at school, university, conferences and at career interviews and recruitment processes. However, McCarthy and Hatcher (2002) suggest that having to make a presentation or speak in public constitutes one of the greatest fears we all face. This is why it is important to be aware of and to develop the techniques and methods of presenting yourself and of preparing an effective presentation as a key study and transferable skill. In this chapter you will learn about some of the keys to preparing, planning and delivering an effective presentation, which might help to overcome some of your fears. Having increased your confidence there is then no substitute for practice.

THE THREE Ps: PREPARATION, PLANNING AND PRACTISE

The three Ps are general principles that you need to use in the lead-up to delivering your presentation. They are applicable in all situations where you will be presenting something to an audience, either as an individual or as part of a group. By following these guidelines, you will have a head start in approaching the task and should feel less nervous and more confident as you will be well prepared for most circumstances.

1. Preparation

Who are you speaking to?

The first thing you need to consider is who you will be speaking to. This is crucial in deciding how to focus your presentation. For example, you may prepare a presentation about caring for stroke patients for your tutor and fellow students as part of an assessment. However, your approach would be completely different if you were to do a similar presentation to a group of unknown health professionals as part of a seminar or conference.

Also bear in mind equality and diversity issues such as gender, disability and cultural differences. Try getting a general idea of who will be in your audience beforehand.

Activity

Think about a group you might have to do a presentation for. Consider the possible profile of your audience taking into consideration issues relating to equality and diversity. How do you make you presentation as inclusive as possible?

What are you talking about?

What are the learning outcomes you are hoping to achieve for your audience and what do you want your audience to do or remember as a result of your presentation? Have you been given a clear brief beforehand? If so you need to ensure you are working closely to this. This will give you the key focus for your presentation and help you identify what might need to be included.

Gathering relevant data

Having decided who you are speaking to and what your key learning outcomes will be, you should gather all the relevant data you will need to ensure you know your subject thoroughly. Preparation for presentation or speech should be the same as for any piece of research such as an essay, assignment or dissertation. Give yourself time to do a thorough literature review, exploiting the range of information sources such as books, journals, quality internet sources and reports. You should reference all sources that you use to back up what you are saying. For more information on this refer to Chapter 1 where Nicola Watkinson explains the literature searching process in detail.

Prepare an outline and KISS

When you feel comfortable with who you are speaking to and what you are going to say you should prepare a basic outline for your presentation. Think about how you might structure what you say to keep your audience interested. Remember that most humans can only concentrate for a maximum of 20 minutes. People respond better to presentations if they are both interested in the topic and involved in the presentation itself, so remember KISS – Keep It Straightforwardly Simple. Do not try to explain huge amounts of theory in ten minutes or read out large blocks of text – you will get lost and confused and your audience will get bored and frustrated. If you can, try to encourage audience participation, either through questions or activities, depending on the circumstances.

Using presentation software such as Microsoft PowerPoint™ can be helpful at this stage, even if you are not going to use it for the presentation itself, as it works on the principle of a series of slides. This allows you to break down what you are going to say into manageable blocks of information, which can be moved around and reworked as you develop the presentation. Of course, you may have your own system for approaching this stage, depending on your personal preferences, such as series of cardboard record cards or using a mind map (see Chapter 4, page 57 for how to create a mind map), so use whatever works best for you.

page 57 for how to create a mind map)

Activity

How would you go about gathering the information for a presentation? You might like to think about a subject you are about to research. Use the information in Chapter 1 of this book to help you do a thorough literature search and then prepare an outline as if you were going to do a presentation. You might like to try this exercise working as a group and decide how you would divide the process up.

Presentations are a two-way process

The best presentations are a learning opportunity for both the audience and the presenter(s). If you are developing your own ideas it is invaluable to enter into a dialogue with the participants. Very often this will be through questions from the audience; it is your choice whether to field questions during your session or to take them at the end. Whatever you decide, make sure you inform the audience at the beginning.

During the preparation stage, you should think about the questions your audience may have about the content of the presentation – and try to answer these during your presentation. Don't worry if you don't think of everything, it is very hard to predict what questions may come up. However, you should be able to prepare for the majority of them, and this is similar to considering what might come up at an interview.

Where will the presentation take place and what equipment will you use?

You need to think about where the presentation will take place as this will help you decide what equipment you might or might not use. If it is in a university lecture theatre or classroom, you will probably have full access to computers, projectors, screens, flip charts, etc. If you are presenting to a community group in a rural village hall you may only have your own voice to rely on, unless you can provide your own equipment. Do not feel pressured into using visual aids and equipment you are unfamiliar with, do what works for you.

It is probably best to imagine the worst-case scenario and work from that point. The worst thing that can happen is that there is a power cut so if you can prepare for your presentation with this in mind you will be ready for anything. Always have notes or handouts for yourself and your audience; at least you will then have a guide as to what you are going to say and something for the audience to follow or to take away.

> **Activity**
>
> Think about a venue in which you might have to give a presentation. See if you can arrange with your tutor to use a suitable room to make this a practical exercise. What equipment will you use? Does it influence how you prepare for your presentation? Does the venue limit you or offer opportunities? What is the worst that could happen and how would you prepare for it?

2. Planning

All forms of communication should have a structure; otherwise your main focus will be lost. Structure is important and you will have already started to develop this in preparing an outline for your presentation. In any public speaking the essential advice is to have a beginning, a middle and an end. In short, say what you are going to say, say it and then say what you have said. Each of these sections carries equal importance and has a clear role to play in the success of your presentation, as you will see.

The beginning

The beginning is crucial. In the first few moments the audience will decide whether they want to listen to you or not. So here are some tips for getting off to a good start.

- Start positively and engage the audience's attention, establishing a relationship with them.
- Don't hide – speak directly to the audience and make eye contact. If you are in a large room try and focus on the middle distance as this will make most people feel you are looking at them.
- Introduce yourself and smile as naturally as possible.
- Introduce your topic and outline what you will be talking about.

- Make each participant feel that you are speaking directly to them and that you want them to learn something new or do something better as a result of your presentation.

The middle

The middle part of your presentation contains the core of what you are going to say and will probably be the longest part. You will find it helpful to break this part down into sections with an understandable sequence and, as in your preparation, you may find presentation software helpful at this stage. Within a 20-minute presentation you will probably only be able to develop a maximum of five clear sections, though the ideal is probably about three. Most public speakers, such as politicians, vicars, etc., will usually have three clear points to get over as this is the most that an audience will probably remember.

It is important to have a clear bridging link between each point and this can either be verbal, for instance, 'I would now like to move on to . . .' or a visual link using presentation software transitions or a simple hand gesture. This will enable you to lead the audience through what you have to say and keep them interested. Try not to labour each point as the audience will lose interest and you risk giving too much emphasis to one section over another.

The end

In the final part of your presentation, you should try to provide a logical conclusion. These are some of the things you should try to do.

- Give a brief summary of what you have said, emphasising the key points.
- Ensure that you make it clear you are finishing; ease into the end, don't just say, '. . . and that's it!' and walk away.
- It is better to begin your conclusion by saying '. . . and now I would like to finish by . . .'
- Thank your audience.
- Don't forget to ask for any questions.
- Ensure that your audience goes away with something in their hands, usually in the form of handouts, to remind them of what you have said.
- Give out evaluation sheets to make sure you get feedback to help you prepare for future presentations.

3. Practise

It is very important that you make time for the third P, practise. Having done the hard work of preparing and planning your presentation it is absolutely essential that you rehearse and practise your performance thoroughly. How you practise is entirely down to personal preference but here are a few suggestions.

- Record yourself reading through the presentation, concentrating on the volume and tone of your voice. This can be an uncomfortable experience as it is always difficult listening to your own voice played back. However, this is what your audience will be listening to.
- Practise the timing of your presentation – are you trying to squeeze too much in? Do you move smoothly between each point?
- Practise with any equipment you might be using, in front of willing volunteers. If you can do this in the venue you will actually be using, all the better.
- If you are using notes make sure that they are not intrusive and that they work for you.
- Learn the introduction to your presentation by heart; this will give you confidence in giving a good first impression.

It is important that you get feedback on your presentation so ask your volunteers to evaluate you. Alternatively, if you have had feedback from presentations you have given previously, use this to fine tune your performance. The following are some points you should consider when you are evaluating your own performance.

- Were my points clear, interesting and in a logical structure?
- Were the pace and volume of the presentation right?
- Did I make a good first impression and was my body language appropriate?
- Did I connect with my audience using direct eye contact, interaction, etc.?
- Were the visual aids I used clear and not intrusive, and did I manage the equipment effectively?
- Was my conclusion handled well?

Sheila Cottrell provides a very helpful self-evaluation sheet, 'How effective am I in giving a talk?' You might want to use this when practising or as a basis for evaluation forms at the end of your presentation (Cottrell, 2003, p. 113).

Use your practise and evaluation to rework your presentation and ensure that all your notes and equipment work for you and you feel comfortable with them. You may still feel nervous but you will certainly be more confident if you give yourself plenty of time to work through the three Ps.

Scenario and Activity

As part of Graham's course assessment he has been asked to do a 20-minute presentation to the course group based on a topic that has been the main focus for the term. He is expected to use media to enhance his presentation where appropriate. Graham has never had to stand up and speak to a group before, or use media such as Microsoft PowerPoint™, although he has had some experience of amateur dramatics. He is fine with researching and writing an assignment but the thought of public speaking terrifies him. How would you help Graham prepare for his presentation? Discuss the following in class or with your tutor to clarify your own understanding in the light of the 3Ps of presentation skills.

DELIVERING THE PRESENTATION

So now the day of your presentation has arrived. Here are some guides to harnessing your performing edge, making a good impression, considering your vocal performance, controlling body language and using media and equipment.

Harnessing your performing edge

It is quite normal to feel nervous when you are about to do something important and potentially challenging. As Andrew Bradbury suggests, you can use this to your advantage by harnessing your performing edge (Bradbury, 2000). If you do not feel a certain amount of anxiety before your presentation, whatever the situation, then there is probably something wrong or you may be more unprepared than you thought. If you have followed the three Ps and given yourself plenty of preparation and practice time then you can go into the performance feeling confident. However, here are a few tips.

- Use relaxation techniques if they help you, such as breathing exercises, t'ai chi, yoga, meditation or just sitting quietly. McCarthy and Hatcher offer a useful relaxation exercise you might like to try (McCarthy and Hatcher, 2002, pp. 50–51).
- It is probably not a good idea to go on a wild night out on the evening prior to your performance. Using drugs, alcohol and other substances just before you go on is definitely not a good idea. This can be challenging if you have been asked to speak following a conference dinner, but try and be restrained.
- The main tool you will be using during this exercise will be your voice, so try some warm-ups. Van Emden and Becker offer some helpful vocal exercises in their book (van Emden and Becker, 2004, pp. 8–9).
- Dress smartly but make sure that you are comfortable as tight and restrictive clothes and shoes won't help you to relax.

Making a good first impression

Now you are confident and as relaxed as possible it is time to walk on. It is important that you present yourself well; this doesn't mean you have to wear a suit, but it is helpful if you dress appropriately for the situation. Walk on confidently and smile if you can, make eye contact and you will form a rapport with your audience more quickly. The presentation begins from the moment you stand up.

It is important to stand during your presentation as this will help you feel more confident, keep you alert and will allow you to project your voice more effectively. Remember that you should not try to hide; you are the main focus for the length of your presentation and anything else will be a distraction. Before you begin check that everyone can see and that they can all hear you. Try not to block any screens or flip charts that you are using and avoid extravagant body language before you begin. As noted above it is helpful if you can memorise the introduction to your presentation, this will get you off to a good start and help your confidence levels.

Your voice

Hopefully, you will have learned to use your voice appropriately while practising your presentation. However, it is all too easy to forget this in the first anxious moments of standing up to begin. So remind yourself of some useful tips.

- Breathe slowly – it is easy to forget to breathe in the heat of the moment.
- Be aware of your volume – you should look up and raise your eyebrows; this will help you to speak up. If you keep your head down you will probably mumble and the audience won't hear you.
- Don't shout – speak audibly and clearly. If you are asked to use a microphone make sure it works and that you hold or place it correctly and don't let it distract you. Van Emden and Becker provide a 'Voice Checklist' that you may find useful (van Emden and Becker, 2004, p. 6).
- The tone of your voice is important – if you speak in a monotone you will lose your audience's attention very quickly. If you smile you are more likely to sound enthusiastic and engaging. This doesn't come naturally to many of us and you will need practice.
- Focus on the normal pace of your speech. Try not to speak too slowly as this will labour your performance and the audience will lose interest. If you are too fast, what you say will not be understood and the audience will miss your key points.
- Avoid slang, jargon and colloquialisms. Assume that you need to explain any technical language unless you are sure that your audience will all understand.
- Avoid using jokes, they rarely work. If you need to use humour do it appropriately and don't force it. In this way it can be useful in keeping your audience's attention.
- Many people worry about 'drying up' – if this happens you should pause and take a few moments to find your place and regroup.

Body language

We all use body language in our everyday communication but it is important to control your non-verbal communication while you are doing your presentation, but without making yourself feel too restricted. Here are a few useful tips.

- Be aware of your gestures and don't fidget – waving your arms wildly or pointing at the projector screen can be very distracting.
- It is fine to move around but don't pace up and down as this can often show that you are anxious.
- You can use a prop such as a pen or a handout as it might keep your hands occupied. However, if you are nervous, any papers you are holding will shake, or you might be tempted to hide behind them and you may start to fidget with your pen. So it might be better if you can go hands free.

- Don't keep your hands in your pockets or slouch, it looks very unprofessional.

Activity

Think of a topic as a group – make it something you are all interested in – and allow each person one minute to do a presentation on that topic. Prepare and plan a brief outline and structure and then do the presentation in front of the group. Get them to give you positive critical feedback on how you performed, paying particular attention to your voice, body language and first impressions. How did you feel, did you use any techniques to harness your performing edge?

Using presentation software and other media and equipment to enhance your presentation

The use of presentation software, such as Microsoft PowerPoint™, for all types of presentation is almost ubiquitous. This means there is a lot of pressure to use the software for any presentation that you may be asked to do. Although it is helpful to be able to use presentation software, it does not mean that you always have to use it, or any other equipment, unless it actively enhances what you have to say and doesn't act as a diversion or distraction. Often, if you are giving a short presentation, it is more powerful if you can feel confident enough to speak directly to your audience without visual aids, as this is more immediate.

However, if you do need to use presentation software make sure that you have all the equipment available to you. You will usually need a laptop or PC (with appropriate software loaded) linked to a projector with a screen to project on to. You may also require speakers linked to the PC or laptop if you are going to use sound clips or music clips. If you wish to demonstrate a live website, you will also need an internet link, although be warned that live online demonstrations don't always go to plan and add an unwelcome risk to your presentation if you are already feeling nervous.

There is not enough space here to go into the detail of getting started with presentation software, although, if you already use word processing software, you will find it quite easy to use. The main difference is that presentation software works on the principle of a series of slides into which you can insert text, images, movie clips, etc. and you can animate the slides and the transition between them. It is particularly useful for:

- presenting images, graphs, diagrams and video clips, but only if they add value to what you are saying and if they are well timed to keep your audience's attention;
- helping to organise, structure and pace your presentation effectively, a slide at a time, in bite-size chunks that the audience can take in;
- helping to prompt you in what you intend to say – if you feel confident enough you might be able to dispense with copious notes and be prompted by each slide;
- printing notes with each slide for your own reference and handouts for the audience that include each slide and a space for notes.

If you decide to use presentation software here are some useful tips to bear in mind:

- use the 6, 7, 8 rule – no more than 6 lines to a slide, letters no less than 7 mm high (about 28 to 32 point), no more than 8–10 slides for a 10-minute presentation;
- check your spelling on all slides;
- be consistent, using the same font and background throughout if possible – remember that using coloured text can be visually disastrous and black on white is too harsh for many people to read, so try to use clear black text, preferably Arial or a sans serif font, on a pastel coloured background;
- don't be too creative with pictures, sounds and animations – many people who discover presentation software for the first time use all the gadgets available – always use them sparingly and only if they emphasise a point, otherwise they are very distracting;
- remember to pause between each slide or as you reveal each line of text or image – if you are rushing to get through the slides you have too many and you need to reduce the number;
- don't put more than one idea on each slide, or try to squeeze too much in, you can always use additional slides if necessary;
- take a look at some examples of other people's presentations on websites such as **www.slideshare.net**.

Presentation software is not the only thing you can use to enhance your presentation. You can use whiteboards (interactive or otherwise), blackboards and flip charts and write comments on them from the audience to introduce some activity and allow everyone to participate. In some venues you may need to use overhead projectors and you can prepare the transparencies using presentation software. In some circumstances you might want to introduce music or soundtracks to create an atmosphere, but be careful what you choose and don't use your presentation to promote your favourite rock band. Music needs to be carefully judged. Whatever tools you use, the most important element is you and what you have to say.

Activity

Find out what equipment might be available to you. Try and practise using presentation software and a range of other equipment and interactive techniques so that you become familiar with them, if you haven't already done so. If possible, incorporate them into some of the exercises mentioned above.

Summary

- Preparation – who are you speaking to? What are you talking about? Where will your presentation take place?

- Prepare an outline and Keep it Straightforwardly Simple (KISS).

- Planning – have a clear structure with a beginning, a middle and an end.

- Practise – allow plenty of time to rehearse and refine your presentation.

- When you are delivering your presentation make sure you harness your performing edge and make a good first impression.

- Be aware of your voice and body language.

- Only use presentation software and other media when it enhances what you have to say.

8

Time Management and Making Good Use of Feedback

Peggy Murphy

Learning outcomes

In this chapter you will learn how to:

- assess which are the best times to study;

- establish how you currently spend your time;

- complete a study plan;

- make use of feedback to improve percentage grades;

- organise your time, to give youself a better chance of success.

INTRODUCTION

Scenario

Sally had to begin to think about preparing for her first assignment. She had a 3 000-word essay to write on communication but she had very little idea about where to begin planning her essay. What would you suggest was the best way for Sally to begin the process of essay writing? Discuss the following chapter with your class or tutor to clarify your own understanding.

Studying on your own can be the most difficult time on the course. This is because there is no structure or system to follow. It is often only when you have given yourself time to develop a systematic approach to studying that you can stop procrastinating and get on with your course work (Northledge, 1994). Many students find that the two main problems that prevent them from progressing on their course are finding enough time to study and, when they do, using the time ineffectively.

Learning the skill of time management is critical to academic success. The secret to making this process less painful is learning how to work smarter, not harder (Lewis, 1994). It may be worth remembering that every student gets 24 hours in a day and 168 hours in a week. This resource is available to everyone. It is valuable to consider that time is a 'non-renewable' resource; once spent it cannot be regained. It is also impossible to accumulate time to save up for a rainy day. Whether you decide to spend your hours wisely, or choose to waste your time, you will still be allocated the same 168 hours per week as everyone else (Payne and Whittaker, 2000).

Mason-Whitehead and Mason (2008) remind us that we have all met people who are well organised, those who appear to sort out everything with consummate ease, planning every meticulous detail from immaculately clear desks. We also know people who appear to be totally devoid of organisational skills. These people often appear to be in a constant state of panic. They are the ones with mounds of paperwork cluttering up their writing surface, who often have difficulty finding anything. It is worth considering your own tendencies and whether you resemble one extreme more than the other, or whether you fluctuate between the two.

Whether you are an organised student or not, most of us have commitments other than study that take up our time. These can be social and family commitments such as childcare or visiting parents. Many students find they need paid work to finance their studies, and some have leisure commitments such as being part of a sports team. When embarking upon a course of study you often have to make choices about how to spend your time and quite often this means giving something up in your life. This can place great strain on your existing relationships, as the time needed for study has to be created from somewhere (Mason-Whitehead and Mason, 2008). The time created is often at the expense of some of the things that you enjoy doing (Maslin-Prothero, 2002). The type of things given up can be nights out with friends or reading for pleasure. However, it is crucial to realise that all work and no play makes for a very dull life. Therefore, it is useful to allocate some time to both the things and the people that you care about, as well as your study.

WORK/LIFE BALANCE

The key is to try to get the balance right between study and all of your other competing activities. It is important to avoid doing so much study that all of your other activities suffer. Conversely, doing so little study that you cannot meet your course commitments is not a great idea (Payne and Whittaker, 2000; Maslin-Prothero, 2002). Also, it can be just as tiring if you do no work all day, as you cannot justify giving yourself a break. It is desirable to maintain a good work/life balance throughout not only your studies but also your career and life. This helps to ensure you achieve both success and happiness. Being realistic about the time you are prepared to devote to your studies will maximise your chances of achieving your goals. If you set unrealistic targets and fail to live up to them, you can start to feel overwhelmed and you could lose confidence in your ability to study (Maslin-Prothero, 2002; Mason-Whitehead and Mason, 2008). Managing your time effectively will reduce stress and improve self-confidence (Payne and Whittaker, 2000). When planning your time it is worth considering that it is both healthy and realistic to accept that you cannot do everything at once. Before you start it is often useful to ask yourself a number of questions.

Activity (Drew and Bingham, 2001; Maslin-Prothero, 2002)

Assess your best times and places to study by completing the following questionnaire.

1. When do you do your best work, is it early morning or late evening?
2. Where do you work most effectively, at home or in the library?
3. What times are you most likely to be able to study undisturbed?
4. Do you study better alone or with others? If you study better with others, who in particular?
5. What circumstances help you study? Do you need peace and quiet, background music, calm, pressure or chocolate?
6. How many hours are you planning to study each week?
7. When are you going to do most of your work? For example, do you propose to work each evening so that you can have your weekends free, or vice versa?

Try not to worry if you don't know how to answer these questions. You many need to find out more about your study habits before you can even begin to plan your time better. When you have answered these questions, begin a week's logbook (Northledge, 1994) to see exactly how you spend each day of your current working/studying week. This will enable you to see where you can find acceptably-sized periods for study within your current weekly schedule.

Activity

How do you fill your 24 hours? Use one of the faces to indicate how you feel about each activity. 😊 😮 😵 ☹ 😣

Date	Time	Activities	Face
	01.00–03.00		
	03.00–05.00		
	05.00–07.00		
	07.00–09.00		
	0900–11.00		
	11.00–13.00		
	13.00–15.00		
	15.00–17.00		
	17.00–19.00		
	19.00–21.00		
	21.00–23.00		
	23.00–01.00		

The exercise in this activity is not as easy as it looks because life is a messy business and does not always divide neatly into the allocated two-hour slots. However, although this is not a straightforward exercise, it can be useful to help you to produce a workable plan of action, instead of simply ambling along (Northledge, 1994). When you have completed the first two activities in this chapter you can then start working on your study timetable and write a 'have to, ought to and like to' do list (see the next activity).

Activity (Payne and Whittaker, 2000)

Have to do	Ought to do	Like to do

This list is designed to help you to prioritise your life. This will help you to determine which areas of your life are important to you, such as relaxation, and which areas, such as household chores, could be delegated to another to make way for study time. Some students write a daily 'to do' list using this 'have to, ought to, like to' principle to enable them to prioritise their day. When you organise your activities you will, in turn, reduce your stress (Payne and Whittaker, 2000). In transition times such as starting a new course at university, it is easy to let the key areas of your life get out of balance, so good time management skills will help to focus your mind on giving sufficient time to the essentials. Following on from the last activity there are a number of revision questions for you to answer in the next activity. These are designed to help you further refine your time management skills.

Activity (Cottrell, 2003)

Why am I doing this course?	
How can I make this as enjoyable as possible?	
Can I make this more interesting?	
Do I do things systematically?	

Are my goals realistic?	
How will I reward myself for meeting my goals?	
Do I eat/sleep/take breaks and relax enough?	
Do I concentrate on improving one aspect of my study and leave others for another day?	
Am I comfortable in my study space?	
Is there enough light/ventilation?	
Am I studying at the best time?	
Do I prioritise before starting to study?	
Do I put off starting my studies (for example, first I need to paint my nails, sort out my sock drawer)?	
Am I aware of my weak points such as making a 'quick' phone call?	
Do I take steps to prevent distractions?	
Could I use distractions, for example, by asking visitors to help?	

TIME WASTERS AND HOW TO COMBAT THEM

It is usual to experience writer's block – this is a normal part of the learning process. These dry spells provide time for you to recharge your batteries, so look upon them as 'fallow' spells. During these times, ideas often quietly percolate in the background. 'Time out' can be necessary to promote new growth and help to synthesise concepts. Sometimes the penny drops when we are doing something completely different from study. It is important to realise that when the 'fallow' times occur it is necessary to honour the time it takes to go through them. With a little luck, you will come out at the other side a bit wiser. It is also vital, however, to recognise when, on a scale of activity, 'time out' changes from being a positive part of the study continuum and moves into the range of becoming a complete waste of time (Payne and Whittaker, 2000).

Procrastination

Everyone is tempted to put off tasks that are boring, difficult or disagreeable. Possible solutions to counter this problem are:

- setting deadlines and sticking to them;
- using prompts so you do not forget;
- promising yourself a reward when you have completed the task;
- breaking an overwhelming task down into bite-sized chunks to make it more manageable.

Perfectionist tendencies

Time is wasted trying to get one element of the project perfect while the other parts suffer. A possible solution to counter this problem is:

- don't try to get it right, just try to get it written – remember that most good essays are written in several drafts before submission.

Poor self-discipline

After committing yourself to study it does not always follow that you will feel like doing the work. Possible solutions to counter this problem are:

- remember that it is often the thought of work, rather than doing the work that is the problem;

- set yourself short tasks of about half an hour to get your motivation up and remember to treat yourself when you have managed to work when you did not feel up to it.

Anxiety

Many students feel overwhelmed at times by the amount of work they have to undertake. Possible solutions to counter this problem are:

- remembering that your time would be better spent by applying yourself to the work, rather than wasting your energy by worrying. If you keep yourself busy, there will not be as much time to worry;
- sharing your anxieties with others – talking to your fellow students and tutors can help to alleviate your anxiety;
- seeking professional help if your worries become serious – your General Practitioner, or a counsellor if your college has one, may be able to offer support.

Poor organisation

If you are untidy and unable to find your things easily, you will waste time before you begin studying. If you get easily distracted, you will waste time. Possible solutions to counter this problem are:

- tidy up every time you finish studying and round off by putting your things away;
- keep your focus on one thing at a time;
- finish one task before starting a new one.

Over-commitment

This often happens to people who cannot say no. Possible solutions to counter this problem are:

- think about fulfilling your own needs as well as everyone else's;
- think about the long-term rewards of being able to say no, such as a successful career or a better grade;
- if you are asked to go out, for example, inform the person who is inviting you that you are too busy right now, but offer an alternative time that suits your plans, such as the weekend;
- make a commitment to yourself to value your time.

Inability to prioritise

Do you find it difficult to concentrate upon the important tasks and get sidelined by trivial things? A possible solution to counter this problem is to complete a weekly 'have to, ought to and like to' do list.

Suggestions to help you deal with some external time wasters

The telephone

When you study you can use caller display or turn the ring tone off. You do not have to answer calls (remember that you are busy). Put the answering machine on. If you decide to answer, let people know you will call them back, or get someone else to answer and take a message.

Visitors

Be polite but firm. Let visitors know what times are convenient for them to call.

Television

The average number of viewing hours in the United Kingdom ranges between 3.3 hours per person per day to 4.2 hours per day. This means that people watch up to a staggering 29.4 hours per week, or 1 528.8 hours per year (Ofcom, 2006). If this is one of the biggest 'thieves' of your free time, allocate yourself viewing time according to the type of programme or set a viewing schedule for each day. Do not watch more than you have allocated. Once you have watched your programme, switch off the television and go back to your studies.

Travelling

If you have to travel by train or bus then why not take a book with you. If you are driving, you could listen to relevant podcasts on your MP3 player or to tapes and CDs on your particular subject while you are in the car.

Socialising

College years are often the best years of your life for socialising but try not to overdo it. For example, you could limit nights out to after 9 p.m. and study for two hours before getting ready to go out. Or you could choose one set night each week to go out and stick to it.

Crises

Some crises are beyond our control and others are self-generated through poor time management. One of my old lecturers had a notice written on their door which read: 'YOUR POOR TIME MANAGEMENT DOES NOT CONSTITUTE A "CRISIS" ON MY BEHALF'.

Activity

1. Think about any ways that you waste time. What are your ideas to solve these problems?
2. What would the consequences be if you implemented those solutions?

Working backwards from deadlines

When you are formulating a plan to write an assignment it can be helpful to work backwards from the final deadline (Drew and Bingham, 2001; Cottrell, 2003). For example:

- deadline for essay, 8 April 2008;
- final draft will be completed by 4 April 2008;
- third draft completed by 28 March 2008;
- second draft completed by 21 March 2008;
- first draft completed by 14 March 2008;
- literature search completed by 7 March 2008 (see Chapter 6 on literature searching).

Activity	How long will it take?	Personal deadlines	How long it really took
Brainstorm/formulate a plan.			
First tutorial.			
Gather information.			
Reading and understanding.			
Organising the information.			
Selecting what to include/leave out.			
Improving first draft.			
Improving second draft.			
Second tutorial.			
Improving third draft.			
Writing up references.			
Writing the final draft.			
Proofreading and editing.			
Final deadline.			

CREATE YOUR OWN POSITIVE LEARNING ENVIRONMENT

If possible, designate a study area in your home (Cottrell, 2003; Maslin-Prothero, 2002; Northledge, 1994). If you do not have a desk or table, use a shelf, storage box or cupboard to keep all of your equipment together. It is advisable to work near to a window that is either behind or to one side of you in order to cut down on distractions. Try to sit on a comfortable chair. Keep your study area tidy and organised; make it somewhere that is inviting to return to.

Suggested study toolkit (Cottrell, 2001)

- Books from the essential book list (bought or obtained from library).
- A4 lined punched paper.
- A4 ring binders for each subject.
- Plastic pockets.
- Small folder for current work – use file dividers to separate contents by subjects.
- Personalise a notebook for your reflective journal.
- Dictionary.
- Thesaurus.
- Calculator.
- Address book for references.
- Diary/Time planner/wall chart.
- Pens, pencils, rubber, coloured pencils, highlighters, stapler, scissors, felt tips, ruler and correction fluid.
- Something to make you smile, such as a plant, photo, poster or joke. If you are going to spend your time studying it is important to create a space that you like being in.

WHAT IS FEEDBACK?

Feedback is central to education. It enables students to maximise their potential throughout their course. Tutors give feedback to students to create an awareness of both their strengths and any areas for improvement. Good feedback highlights how students can improve their performance. Throughout your programme of study you will be given feedback from your tutors.

Making use of feedback

If you are concerned about submitting your work, particularly if it is for the first time, be assured that you are not alone. One of the main concerns that students face is putting their work forward for scrutiny. Tutors recognise the importance of offering an honest appraisal of students' work against maintaining students' confidence in their ability to complete the course (Norman and Hyland, 2003). The comments that lecturers make are designed to help you improve and develop your ability while on the course. Lecturers spend a considerable amount of time assessing work and writing feedback and the main reason for this is to ensure that students benefit from this process (Lloyd, 2007). One of the crucial aspects of assessing work in higher education is to motivate students to take responsibility for their own learning (Regan, 2003). The Higher Education Funding Council for England (HEFCE, 1995) recommends that one way tutors can facilitate this is to provide students with feedback that is both timely and detailed.

When encouraging an environment of autonomous learning, tutors are aware that feedback is an essential part of this process. Formative (informal feedback designed to develop you) and summative (feedback that is marked) assessments are offered throughout the student's experience. This feedback impacts upon students' learning. The way that feedback is presented can have a marked effect on creating a positive student learning environment. Giving criticism is essential in order to aid development but, when highlighting students' weaknesses, it is vital not simply to identify them but to suggest ways in which the student can improve their work. Therefore, beginning and ending on a positive note is recommended to increase confidence in students (Fry *et al.*, 2003). Tutors need to give feedback to students in order for the students to improve their performance. Tutors may fail to give constructive feedback on occasion. If this occurs then it is your responsibility as an adult student to ask them to comment upon the strengths you can build on as well as acknowledge the areas for improvement. Good tutors will always offer advice on how to improve your work but it is up to you whether you heed their advice.

Activity

Look at the following assignment feedback sheet and work out what the student needs to do to improve their grade.

Assignment feedback sheet (health studies)

Course: Pre-registration (Fitness for Practice)
Name: **A Student**
Level: **6**
Assignment title: NUR 366

Submission date: 30 July 2007

Section 1	Section 2	Section 3	Section 4	Section 5	Total	Grade
15%	30%	35%	10%	10%		
8	15	22	8	7	60	B

Comments:
Thank you for your work which was of a good standard. Although your introduction signposted most of your answer you did not specify which management issue out of the four stated on the brief that you would address. It was not until page 4 that the educative role of the nurse was alluded to. You provided a good discussion around oral hygiene; you could have linked this to the management issue more closely, for example discussing how audits may ascertain the extent of the problem. On page 8 you discuss quality assurance; again this was not mentioned in your introduction. You provided a good discussion which demonstrated your knowledge of the subject. Your section on change, although well researched, could have been structured better to make your essay flow more easily. The conclusion was well written and pulled your assignment together.

The main areas of improvement are:
- to ensure you signpost every aspect of your answer in the introduction (you could have mentioned each of your subheadings).
- you could work on linking themes together and synthesising the knowledge you have gained.

That said, this was a good analytical piece of writing which demonstrated your ability to evaluate research and nursing literature. Well done, A Student.

What to do after you have received feedback

- Read and reread all of your tutor's comments.
- If you still need some guidance and clarity, make an appointment to discuss the feedback with your tutor.
- If you are disappointed with your mark and feedback, be kind to yourself. Have a bubble bath, a pint with friends or whatever you do to unwind. Then give yourself a day or two to reflect before making an appointment to see your tutor. Look at your own SWOT analysis (see Chapter 11 on CVs and Interviews) to remind yourself that you (like everyone else) have strengths as well as weaknesses.

REVISION QUIZ

1. How many hours are there in a week?

2. Define the term 'work/life balance'.

3. Name two advantages of managing your time effectively.

4. What should you do if you have a 'dry spell' in your studies?

5. What should you do if you feel overwhelmed or anxious about studying?

6. What are the average TV viewing times per day/year?

7. What does working backwards from a deadline entail?

8. How does feedback benefit your education?

9. What can you do to make the most of feedback?

10. How will you keep yourself motivated throughout your course?

Profiles and Portfolios

Chris O'Grady

Learning outcomes

This chapter will:

- provide an insight into what profiles and portfolios are;

- provide an understanding of the purpose of a portfolio;

- provide guidance on constructing a portfolio;

- provide an insight into how reflective practice helps to demonstrate learning.

INTRODUCTION

This chapter will provide you with the necessary knowledge and guidance to compile your own 'profile' or 'portfolio'. The aim of the chapter is to deliver an introduction to the ideas behind profile and portfolio construction and to strengthen your knowledge and understanding about why they are needed. Additionally, this chapter will give you some helpful pointers for creating a profile or portfolio and it will help to make the process easier for you. It is important to clarify that the terms 'profile' and 'portfolio' tend to be used interchangeably in health and social care.

PROFILES OR PORTFOLIOS – WHAT DO THESE TERMS MEAN?

There appears to be much confusion about how the differing use of the terms has arisen. The way that the terms are used appears to relate to the purpose of the profile or portfolio. The term often associated with the accreditation of prior experiential learning (APEL) is portfolio preparation. The APEL portfolio is designed to show prior learning in the context of the course upon which the student wishes to embark (Nganasurian, 1999). More recently, the concept of a portfolio has developed within professional practice in terms of providing evidence of the practitioner's competence and continuing development. Thus, there has been a movement away from the use of the portfolio as merely a record of things that have happened towards its evolvement as a continuously changing artefact that is used for learning (Jasper, 2003).

Mason-Whitehead and Mason (2008) define a portfolio as a body of work that is put together by the student over a period of time, demonstrating the student's ability and learning achievements. Similarly, Hull *et al.* (2005) sum up a portfolio as being a way of enabling the student to keep a record of their personal and professional development, their professional experiences and qualifications. Brown (1992) is one of the few authors to differentiate the terms, defining a profile as a collection of evidence that is selected from the personal portfolio for a particular purpose and audience. The majority, however, would advise that it is best not to get too hung up over which term you decide to adopt. A profile or a portfolio is a dynamic and positive means of demonstrating that you are developing knowledge and competence, and encouraging the engagement in lifelong learning.

Whatever term is used, the principles of keeping a profile or portfolio are generally the same for all professionals. To avoid confusion for the remainder of the chapter the term portfolio will be used.

Activity

Take five minutes to think about what the purpose of a portfolio might be. Think about the benefits both to yourself and your audience (the person who will be reading it).

WHAT PURPOSE DOES A PORTFOLIO SERVE?

As a professional, having up-to-date evidence of the type of experiences and learning that you have encountered is a powerful means of demonstrating your professionalism and competence. Developing the portfolio helps to link understanding about clinical experience and theoretical knowledge within a discipline. It provides opportunity to create self-awareness, recognise and develop your potential and build on your confidence in relation to your practice and educational capabilities. Displaying your achievements and progress in this way can assist you in gaining educational or employment opportunities. The main benefits of constructing a portfolio include:

- providing up-to-date evidence of achievements and qualifications;
- creating an awareness of learning and life experiences;
- encourages personal and professional development;
- encourages reflective practice;
- encourages the delivery of evidence-based practice.

HOW WILL THE PORTFOLIO BE ASSESSED?

Institutions tend to differ in their approach to the assessment of portfolios. While some will include them as part of the student's assessment process, others will not require them to be part of the formal assessment, using them solely as a vehicle to facilitate student learning.

PLANNING THE PORTFOLIO

Different formats will suit different individuals so this section is intended as a guide to support the process rather than to dictate exactly how a portfolio has to be completed.

Activity

Take five minutes to think about what you might need to consider when planning your portfolio.

What do you need to consider when planning your portfolio?

Before starting to compile your portfolio it is important to consider the following.

- Decide what you are willing to disclose, because other people such as potential employers or personal tutors will be reading your portfolio.
- Consider the time frame for completion.
- Think about why you have to complete a portfolio.

If you are developing your portfolio to gain access to employment or an educational course, you will need to complete the work by a set deadline. It is a good idea to set yourself a plan as to what you can realistically achieve on a weekly or monthly basis. Whatever the purpose is for compiling a portfolio, you will more than likely have a set time frame in which to complete the work. Setting yourself deadlines for planning and achieving certain aspects of the work will help to keep you focused and foster a healthy work/life balance. Remember that the worst thing to do is to leave your work until the last minute because an unforeseen situation might occur that prevents you from carrying out the work to your best ability. (See Chapter 8 for more information on how to plan your work).

Take time to think about why you have to compile a portfolio and who will be reviewing the documentation. This way, you will ensure that the information links appropriately and the claims that you make about your knowledge and skills are recognised. Think about how to ensure that there is sufficient evidence to demonstrate the learning that has taken place and how the knowledge you have gained will impact on your future practice.

How do I compile the portfolio?

Some students will need to develop their profile from scratch and others will be provided with formatted pages, complete with a binder. The portfolio tends to be constructed for a particular purpose, as opposed to having free content decided by the student. Nevertheless, whatever type is needed, it will require careful planning. At the beginning of your course or programme of study, if a portfolio is required you will normally be given clear advice about how it needs to be compiled. This should include advice on how to edit the material to prevent the portfolio from becoming too large and unworkable. The material included should be relevant, clear, concise and coherent.

PORTFOLIO PRESENTATION

The main criterion is that the portfolio should be neat, look professional, have a clear logical flow, with the different pieces of evidence being easy to locate. The work should be well presented, legible, accurate and grammatically correct. The following points provide some helpful tips on how to achieve this.

- Make a contents page so that the information is easy to locate.
- Insert dividers between each section.
- You may wish to word process the work so that it is neat and easy to read.
- Present the information in an orderly manner.
- Use the same style and format throughout.
- Think about the picture it will be presenting – take pride in the work as it is a representation of you and your professionalism, view it as an opportunity to 'sell' yourself when applying for future employment opportunities.

WHAT GOES INTO A PORTFOLIO?

The portfolio may include information such as a CV (see Chapter 11), details of clinical work placements, learning contracts, tutorials and reflective accounts. Reflection tends to play a significant part of portfolio development and will be explored in more depth later in the chapter. To make the task easier to understand, Jasper (2003) suggests that, when you are compiling a portfolio, you should compare the process to producing a family photograph album. When you are choosing from all the photographs that you have, you select those that present the best possible picture of you. You are unlikely to want to show others unflattering photos or any that you would be embarrassed about. Similarly when you are selecting the documentation for your portfolio, it is just as important to create a good picture of yourself in this way.

Activity

To help you compile your portfolio, ask yourself the following questions:

1. What past work experiences or training do I have?
2. What life experiences do I have?
3. What have I learned from these experiences?
4. Which of this learning is relevant to this course?
5. What does it say about me as a person/professional?

Figure 1 is an example of the type of material that may be incorporated in your portfolio.

Section 1 Personal profile.	• Educational background. • Work experience. • Student biography.
Section 2 Self-assessment and action plans.	• SWOT Analysis – Strengths, Weaknesses, Opportunities and Threats. • Plan of future learning.
Section 3 Practical placements.	• Student/mentor contracts. • Appraisal of personal performance. • Record of practice hours.
Section 4 Reflections.	• Reflections on practical experience.
Section 5 Assessments.	• Record of student's marks.
Section 6 Tutorials.	• Record of meetings with personal tutor and/or mentor. • Assignment guidance/feedback.
Section 7 Learning outcomes.	• Learning objectives/methods of achievement.

Figure 1 Example of the components of a portfolio

Personal profile

This section should provide the reader with an overview of your past experience. Remember to include both personal and professional details. This may include the following:

- personal details;
- general education;
- further education/higher education;
- employment history;
- qualifications;
- courses attended;
- hobbies;
- life skills;
- personal and professional aspirations.

It is likely that the person reading your work does not know you or have any idea as to your academic or practice ability. Providing the above information will introduce you to the reader and inform them of past achievements and your future goals and aspirations.

Self-assessment and action plans

Self-assessment plans help to appraise your performance and experience to date. They can relate to areas of your professional or personal life that have had an impact on your learning and the knowledge that has been gained. Taking the time to complete the self-assessment will help to keep your learning focused and assist you in planning how to get the most out of future learning opportunities. The self-assessment plan and action plan interlink as, once you have identified your learning needs, developing an action plan helps you to decide how you will meet those needs. Self-assessment is a continuous process. Therefore, it is important to reappraise your performance in preparation for each practice experience that you have planned. At the end of the placement you should take time to evaluate whether or not the goals that you had planned for yourself are achieved or still need to be worked on. One way of helping you to do a self-assessment is to carry out what is called a SWOT analysis.

SWOT analysis

This will require identifying your:

- Strengths;
- Weaknesses;
- Opportunities;
- Threats.

A SWOT analysis will help you to think about what your strong points are as well as areas that you need to work on and improve. In addition it will encourage you to consider personal and professional opportunities and what factors may prevent or obstruct you from making the most of these. Carrying out the SWOT analysis will help to identify your own learning needs and highlight aspects of your practice that you need to change or develop (see Chapter 11 for more information on developing your SWOT analysis).

Strengths

This gives you the opportunity to draw on the things you are good at. To help, think about what a friend might say your good points are. The strengths can relate to personal or professional aspects of your life. You may wish to focus on some of your achievements to date. This could include qualifications or courses that you have undertaken or the skills you have developed. Personal aspects could relate to your family life, hobbies or any voluntary work.

Weaknesses

When thinking about your weaknesses remember that a weakness does not necessarily mean you are bad at something. We cannot be good at everything, some skills need to be improved or developed further. Again, think about what a colleague might describe as being your weaknesses.

Opportunities

Often we forget to think about what learning opportunities are available to us. Think about the type of practice placement you will be experiencing next and what opportunities this may offer. Your practice mentor can advise you on the type of experiences available to you during the placement and what you need to do to access them.

Threats

What factors may prevent you from achieving what you want to do? Consider if any of the weaknesses you have identified may cause a threat to your learning. The threats could relate to academic work, your practice or personal factors. The next thing you need to do is to think of a strategy to overcome these barriers.

> ### Activity
>
> Try and devise your own SWOT. When doing so think about the type of practice environment and experience you will be encountering next.

Developing your action plan

Focus on all the areas covered in the SWOT. Think about each of the points you have raised in turn; are there any connections between them? Your action plan should consider how you are going to tackle your weaknesses and draw upon your strengths. Think about the future opportunities that are available and how you are going to make use of them. Your action plan must be realistic and represent the areas of practice that you want to concentrate on next. This will help to keep you focused and to build confidence in your abilities.

> ### Activity
>
> Devise your own action plan, incorporating the strategies that you are going to use to help improve your weak areas. Plan what you need to do to get the most out of your next learning experience.

Student/mentor contracts

The student/mentor contract will provide an opportunity for both student and mentor to focus on the learning opportunities available and the potential learning that could occur. It allows the student and mentor to set aside time to negotiate the terms and conditions, along with the responsibilities of each party. Before starting a new practice experience, try and link your SWOT analysis so that it relates to the future learning opportunities and what you are hoping you may be able to achieve during this period of practice. Your mentor will be able to discuss whether or not the skills or areas of practice that you want to experience are realistic and relate appropriately to the stage in your training. At a midway point in your practice placement, the student/mentor contract will provide an opportunity to look at what you have managed to achieve so far, what areas you need to continue to work on and what future opportunities are left to explore. At the end of the practice placement, the final part of the student/mentor contract should allow for overall feedback on your work, attitude, commitment and progress.

Activity

Think about what might be the purpose of setting up a student/mentor contract, and its benefits to your future learning.

The student/mentor contract:

- provides an opportunity to think about the areas of practice you have already developed and what areas of learning are still outstanding;
- provides an opportunity to focus on how you might achieve future learning;
- allows both student and mentor to outline their responsibilities;
- provides an opportunity to discuss progress;
- allows the mentor to detail what has been observed and how the performance criteria and ranges of experience were covered;
- provides the student with opportunity to reflect on their practice and the learning that has been achieved.

Reflection

The aim of this section is to explore ways in which you can incorporate the reflective work that you undertake within your portfolio. Reflection is an ideal vehicle for providing evidence of achievement. Reflection will suit some students and not others, just as some forms of learning have more appeal to us than others. Students often tend to deliberate over what the topic area should be for the reflection. However, it is not necessarily the subject of the reflection that is important, but its analysis in terms of what can be drawn out to demonstrate understanding and learning. The reflective piece will help to show how you are applying your knowledge and the learning that has been gained from the experience in practice.

How do you decide what experience to reflect on?

When you are deciding which experience to reflect on think about the purpose of your reflection and why you are doing it. To help you choose the experiences think about the following:

- the aspects of your practice you feel you do well;
- the aspects of your practice that you have felt happy or proud about;
- the times when you have received recognition;
- the times when you have put in a lot of trouble or effort;
- things that have not gone well;
- the times when you have found an experience negative or disturbing in some way;
- things that make you feel uncomfortable.

What skills do you need for reflection?

Reflection needs thought and preparation. Atkins and Murphy (1992) highlighted that the following skills are needed for reflective practice.

- self-awareness;
- descriptive skills
- critical analysis;
- synthesis;
- evaluation.

Activity

Think about the above skills. Then focus on an experience that happened to you in practice; choose one that has stuck out in your mind. Ask yourself the following questions.

- What did you do?
- Where did you get your knowledge from to do it that way?
- Is there anything that you needed to do differently?
- What new learning occurred and how will you be able to use this in your future practice?

How do you present the reflective account?

There are many reflective models or frameworks that can be used to guide and structure the reflection such as, for example, Gibbs (1998), Johns (2000) or Stephenson (2000). For those who are novices at reflection it is advisable to first read around the models and then select the one which best fits your needs. As you become more experienced at reflection, you may choose not to use a model and you will feel comfortable in presenting the reflection in your own logical format. Unless it is stipulated as part of your programme of study that you use a model it does not really matter, as long as the description of the experience or incident is clearly presented and does not leave the reader to question what was happening, who was involved and what you were trying to achieve. The reflection should outline the main learning that has taken place. Try and make links between the theory and practice elements and analyse why the experience went the way it did. Think about whether there was anything else that needed to be done and what you might do differently in the future. Reflection does not always come easily to students and initially it can feel quite daunting. Reflection, like anything else, becomes easier with practice and experience.

CONCLUSION

A portfolio is seen as a collection of documents that provides a picture to a third party of what a person is like in relation to their educational or professional growth. The portfolio is designed to assist the student to develop and recognise their potential, forming a record of evidence, which monitors personal and professional development. It demonstrates how students progress in both the theoretical and practice elements of the programme. Developing the portfolio requires careful planning and preparation. The way that you present your portfolio will say a lot about your commitment to learning. It is important that the information is presented in a clear, logical manner and looks professional.

Reflection can play an important part in demonstrating students' learning and the ability to link theory to practice. Reflection enables changes to be made to future practice or help the student to establish what future knowledge is required to tackle similar situations more effectively. Carrying out self-assessment or self-appraisal helps you to take stock of your experiences while, at the same time, look towards future personal and professional goals. The learning involved can provide a dialogue between student and mentor/tutor to evaluate strengths and weaknesses, and identify future opportunities and any barriers which need to be overcome. Additionally, the completed portfolio documentation contains all the evidence required to ensure that, on completion of the programme of study, the student is fit for practice, purpose and award (NAfW, 2002). The portfolio may be used as a means of assisting the student to gain access to either employment or future educational opportunities.

Summary

- Profiles and portfolios are tools for demonstrating learning.
- Portfolios are ongoing resources for future personal and professional development.
- Self-assessment and reflection are important parts of portfolio building.
- Portfolios aid individual learning by targeting individual learning needs.

10

Critical Thinking: a Six-stage Process

Tracey Ross

Learning outcomes

By the end of this chapter you will be able to:

- appreciate the rationales for critical thinking;
- understand the process for critical thinking;
- challenge future literature with a more open and questioning mind;
- apply the technique of critical thinking to multiple settings.

INTRODUCTION – AN ETHICAL AND PHILOSOPHICAL APPROACH TO STUDYING

Thinking is one of the most fundamental of human activities. Synthesising new information in order to enhance psychomotor development and social interaction begins at birth. Attention, recognition, labelling and analysing form the building blocks for lifelong learning as humans draw together knowledge from multiple sources in order to inform their daily decision-making. As this form of thinking is central to humanity and practised almost instinctively, one would assume that it would be an effortless process to harness this skill in order to engage in work of academic distinction. Thinking, however, appears to be the student's greatest source of anxiety.

Students are given the freedom and permission to think, which in itself creates problems as educators equate freedom with skill and disposition. Despite the necessity to think on a daily basis, van Gelder (2004) argues that humans are not natural critical thinkers, they are pattern-seeking, story-telling animals, and this results in most academic work being labelled as 'descriptive' rather than critical. Critical thinking is a craft and, like most crafts, it needs engagement, nurture and practise. There is an expectation that, as students engage with theory, comparing and contrasting the various viewpoints will be a natural outcome. However, critical thinking is a purposeful cognitive process and therefore it requires training and development. This is the educator's challenge as education's most crucial mission is to teach students how to think rather than what to think.

The aim of this chapter is to liberate the student's mind by highlighting the basic elements of critical thinking. In doing so this chapter should help the student to enhance their academic and professional confidence.

WHY SHOULD WE THINK CRITICALLY?

Critical thinking is the key to gaining high marks in assignments. This is the student's mission. It is a mistake to equate critical thinking with intelligence as two equally intelligent students may think in very different ways. The intelligent student who applies intellect without critique may achieve the assignment objectives but the student who applies the technique of critiquing will achieve a deeper understanding of those objectives and, through deep sceptical enquiry, will be better able to demonstrate that understanding and, hence, should achieve the higher grade.

Critical thinking is not just about achieving higher grades but is a lifelong transferable skill. It is relevant to every human situation as life is a constant process of learning. Thinking, and the decisions made on the basis of that thinking, impacts on the quality of human life. From birth, humans unconsciously select from a wide range of available options in order to solve daily problems. Raising those options into consciousness and deliberately debating their relevance increases confidence in personal decision-making and confidence in one's own personal character. The application of critical thinking gives students the interpersonal confidence to challenge in a constructive manner in situations outside of the academic context, such as in social situations or in the professional arena, as a wide variety of data types are synthesised. Critical thinking helps to move health and social care forward; innovation can only be an outcome in a climate of thoughtful deliberation. Change has consequences and, as such, should be implemented on the basis of substantive and intellectual reasoning.

Modern health and social care is concerned with the nurture and care of vulnerable people. Therefore, professionals have a moral mandate to provide the highest level of care possible based upon an assessment of individual need – 'one shoe does not fit all'. In order to make informed judgements, professionals need to critically evaluate the range of therapies and solutions available and be selective. Modern health and social care with its governance agenda requires decisions based upon well-founded arguments and reliable evidence. Studies and theories need to be evaluated for their relevance, logic, safety and scientific merit. Vulnerable people deserve this consideration and, furthermore, should professionals not desire to give their best?

WHAT IS CRITICAL THINKING?

In order to enhance understanding it is sometimes easier to illustrate what something is not rather than to describe what it is.

Critical thinking is not criticising

The term 'critic' comes from the Greek and means 'one who discerns or is in a position of disagreement'. It carries very negative connotations, implying that an unfavourable evaluation is given. The inference is that criticism is an opportunity to gripe or fault-find rather than to cultivate intellectual growth. Criticism is a biased analysis that involves one viewpoint to the exclusion of all others, it is subjective and self-focused. It is often used to express negative opinions rather than positive ones. Criticism implies finality and closure whereas critical thinking is concerned with opening the mind and liberating the thinking process. Critical thinking is the starting point of dialogue whereas criticism is the end of the conversation.

Critical thinking is not description

Many students may be familiar with this term and may feel exasperation when the term is used to rationalise a grade that is lower than expected. Description is concerned with telling it like it is; it gives an account of reality from one person's viewpoint, with no support or rationality. Description does not include any explanations for the viewpoint or investigate where the viewpoint originates. Description does not challenge the viewpoint or offer any alternative positions.

Scenario

Mr Richards was a 60-year-old gentleman who entered the clinic carrying a walking stick. He was a small man and spoke in a very soft voice. His wife was a large lady who shouted out the answer each time that her husband was asked a question. It is common for spouses to answer on their husband's behalf, especially in the village of Whivbridge. In Whivbridge, men tend to be short and slim and speak with a soft southern accent.

In this example, the student tells the reader about Mr and Mrs Richards' clinic visit but does not debate or explore any of the information given, such as, why was he carrying a walking stick – is he infirm? Could it belong to his wife? Did he find it outside the clinic and wish to enquire to whom it belongs? There are several options to explore regarding the use of the walking stick. The critical thinker would seek an explanation for the stick by exploring all of the available options and evaluating the rationality of each option, then make an informed judgement based on evidence and logic. The critical thinker will also seek causal links between the size of the man, the soft voice, the accent and the village of Whivbridge. They will evaluate the available evidence to support the links. The critical thinker has an enquiring mind and needs to see more than the presenting picture – as the thinker sees more, they will naturally give more.

Critical thinking is . . .

There are many definitions of critical thinking, most of which include terms such as analysis, evaluation, scepticism, logic, questioning and clarifying. Critical thinking is an objective evaluation about the quality of a piece of work, it evaluates the logic, interpretations, methods, findings and conclusions in order to make informed judgements or solve problems.

Critical thinking involves reading information then pulling that information apart in order to question the logic within it. Basically, it concerns the identification of an overall message; it examines the structure of the message, evaluates the rationality within the message and appraises the strength of the evidence available to support the message. This involves the willingness to examine information from as many sides as possible in order to establish logic and reason. A critical thinker asks questions about beliefs, gathers information, evaluates the information and comes to reliable and trustworthy conclusions about the given message. Becoming a critical thinker is more than applying a given technique, it requires a disposition and a willingness to be open-minded and the discipline to practise.

HOW TO THINK CRITICALLY: A SIX-STAGE PROCESS

Stage one: reading and reflection upon practice

There is no standard model for critical thinking but several authors have tried to propose models such as Mottola and Murphy (2001), Sullivan and Decker (1997) and Edwards (1998). The majority of authors agree that critical thinking requires a raising of awareness and continual practise in order for the process to become normative. The key to critical thinking and writing is critical reading. Close and copious reading is crucial, as one cannot be critical if one does not have options to draw upon; one cannot be selective in the absence of variety. Critical reading requires the reader to focus on and engage with the text in order to question; therefore, finding the correct level of text is fundamental. Many students make the mistake of accessing high-level texts, obscured by jargon, and fail to identify with the theory. It is important to access the level of literature that suits the individual student and then build upon this as understanding progresses and practice develops.

Scenario

A first-level diploma student approached their tutor and stated that they wished to withdraw from a course as they could not comprehend the anatomy and physiology. 'Which texts have you accessed?' asked the tutor. '*Gray's Anatomy*,' replied the student. *Gray's Anatomy* is a high-level textbook commonly used by medical students.

Stage two: identifying the premise

Close reading allows the reader to focus attention on the author's message or premise and to identify the key points in order to make an accurate interpretation (Cottrell, 2005). It involves paying close attention to detail; identifying and separating the relevant from the dross; and sometimes it necessitates repetitive reading. This tends to be more successfully achieved if the reader selects one paragraph at a time and consciously asks, 'What is the author telling me?' Authors can be compared to sales personnel in that each one is trying to sell you their point of view. The uncritical reader is vulnerable to each sales person.

Activity

Try to identify the author's premise in the following text:

A profession without a credible research foundation is doomed and may be deemed a ship on the high seas with a hole in the hull (Ramsden, 2005). Nursing has existed in a research vacuum for many years and occupies the lowest position in the research league tables compared to other professions. Decisions about care have been made on a ritualistic basis rather than being rooted in logic, evidence and innovation. This could be explained by its hand-maiden image and the mandate to do as one is told. Evidence from research studies shows that there is a high percentage of women employed in nursing and it is well known that women do not like to challenge the status quo. For nursing to progress and achieve professional recognition a change in attitude and focus is required, nurses need to perform research to survive.

Which of the following is the author's message?

1. Nursing is about sailing.
2. Nursing is about obeying orders.
3. Compared with other professions, nursing is not performing enough research and its professional status is under threat as a result.
4. Nursing needs more men as there are too many women.

In this example, number 3 is clearly the correct premise; the author wants his audience to believe that nursing is under threat professionally, due to the lack of research undertaken. The author has a particular view about research activity and is trying to persuade the reader of his viewpoint. However, some irrelevant material is also included that could detract from the message and lead the reader down a different path. For example, a student could focus their attention upon the issue of nurses as handmaidens or upon gender issues and completely miss the agenda.

Stage three: scepticism

The most distinctive feature of a good critical thinker is the ability to be sceptical or open-minded. Being open-minded involves having a tolerance for new ideas and divergent views. Cottrell (2005) refers to this stage as holding polite doubt. This stage involves firstly questioning the extent to which the author's premise can be believed. The reader evaluates the extent to which the claims fit with known reality. The reader should therefore ask the following questions.

- Do I believe this?
- If yes, why?
- How does it fit with what I currently understand?
- Who else agrees with this view?
- Is there any additional support?

The reader is looking for rationality in the claims. They should then seek indications as to why the premise should not be believed and look for support. Achieving both of these tasks involves seeking out the various views and positions that exist regarding the issues under discussion and viewing them from as many sides as possible. This can be an unsettling process as often it calls for a period of reflection and introspection and can lead to a change in long-held belief systems as the reader considers viewpoints that contradict their own.

It is important to highlight that critical thinking is not concerned with necessarily seeking truth as one could question the extent to which absolute truths exist. Rolfe (2000) argues that knowledge is not about what we know but about what we believe that we know. Two students' evaluations about a piece of text may differ but may not be wrong. Common-sense understanding is impacted by socialisation, culture exposure, cognitive make-up and self-awareness. Reality is merely a process of interpretation so, if one applies the method of critical thinking, the logic will be unique to that person. There are no right answers, just different ways of seeing things (Carroll, 2004).

Cottrell (2005) suggests that scepticism is not about doubting everything, as humans need to have some trust in the world in order to exist within it. Too much scepticism results in a failure to commit to anything while too little leads to gullibility. Therefore, scepticism involves being selective about the number of messages to investigate as most assignments are constrained by word limits.

For example, if we return to the student activity above, we can apply the principle of scepticism to the author's premise now that it has been identified. Can we believe that the professional status of nursing is under threat due to a paucity of research performed by its members? Making a judgement about the plausibility of this claim will result in the reader needing to investigate the world of nursing. This may start with the reader asking the following questions.

- What do I know about nursing?
- How does this understanding fit with the author's premise?
- How does it support the premise?
- In which ways does it not support the premise?

At this stage, the reader establishes a preliminary logic and either rejects or accepts the premise but this is based upon only one form of understanding and is a biased viewpoint. The reader now needs to look for support or refutation from additional external sources in order to objectify the held belief. This involves searching available literature (see Chapters 1, 4 and 6) and accessing expert viewpoints.

Stage four: arguments and evidence

The extent to which claims can be believed is impacted by the extent to which the author provides support for the viewpoint. In order to be persuasive the writer provides reasons as to why the premise should be believed. Some of these reasons will be rooted in logic and some will be rooted in evidence. Cottrell (2005) refers to these reasons as contributing arguments and states that they provide a case for the premise and are the pillars of the argument. The more pillars, the stronger the case.

If we return to the student activity, we can see that the author is making several premises, one being that nurses do not perform research because they are handmaidens who do as they are told. Therefore, the author is providing a reason for why they do not carry out research. In this way, the author is contributing to the argument and selling the reader the idea. The author is hoping that the reader will buy the argument based on the assumption that they have similar belief systems. However, logic relies upon the assumption that a single reality exists but people are different. Therefore, logic is subjective and not necessarily strong enough to justify a particular premise or position. Evidence is needed.

The hierarchy of evidence

Confusion exists about exactly what constitutes good evidence as Carper (1978) values personal and ethical knowledge whereas Crombie (1996) rejects these as too subjective and only accepts that which can be scientifically proven. McClarey and Duff (1997) suggest that a hierarchy of evidence exists, as identified below.

- A meta-analysis of all randomised control trials concerning a particular topic is considered the best level of evidence.
- Second in the hierarchy is one particularly good experiment about the topic.
- Next, surveys are recognised as having high scientific value, as the results can be generalised to a large number of people.
- Qualitative research that involves performing interviews, observations or focus groups is not as highly regarded, as these involve a smaller number of people.

So far, the hierarchy of evidence is concerned with the actual performance of research studies. Following on from these are written pieces of work, listed in order of credibility.

- a literature review that examines all of the written work available about a topic; these are considered less credible than research as they can include opinion-based work, policy documents and case studies;
- the work of an expert who gives their opinion;
- multiple opinions that agree about a topic but may not be the opinions of experts;
- one opinion-based piece of work – opinion-based work is often referred to as anecdotal and is considered less credible than research as it is more difficult to discover and evaluate the process of logic.

The problem with this hierarchy is that it assumes that science can solve all problems. However, science does not completely explain many facets of reality; for example, religion and the paranormal are rooted in belief rather than prediction and control. Furthermore, sometimes the human brain can get it right, meaning that a person can sometimes arrive at a reliable, valid conclusion without really knowing why or how. Nevertheless, the hierarchy does provide student critical thinkers with a starting point for evaluation. The student should question where the evidence they are using fits within the hierarchy.

Rigour

All studies have strengths and weaknesses and need to be evaluated for their rigour in terms of method, procedure, ethics and theoretical consistency. This requires a basic knowledge of the research process and the disposition to question. Several models exist to assist students with this process, such as Crombie (1996), Cormack (2006) and Cottrell (2005). Most models contain similar criteria and include evaluating the recency of the work, the compatibility between the theory and the methods, the sampling procedures, ethical procedures and analysis of the results. It is considered good practice to use the most up-to-date evidence. However, this does not necessarily mean that a more recent study will be a more rigorous one, hence, several criteria need to be considered.

Quantative or qualitative research

Different types of research require specific types of methods in order to gather the data needed. For example, a type of research termed 'quantitative research' requires large samples of people so tends to adopt surveys rather than interviewing as a method. 'Qualitative' styles of research, on the other hand, seek deep, meaningful information about people's perceptions or experiences and, therefore, adopt more interactive methods such as interviews or focus groups. This compatibility between the type of research and the methods used is fundamental to achieving accurate results, as all the following steps in the process will be invalid if an incongruent approach is used. Validity refers to the extent to which the method or instrument used adequately represents the phenomena under study (Cormack, 2006) or the extent to which it appears to be a true reflection of reality, whereas reliability refers to the extent to which a study can be replicated and achieve the same findings. The evidence is only as good as the search for the data and is only as accurate as that which is available.

Activity

1. Return to the previous activity on page 139 and identify the different types of evidence that exist within it, i.e. anecdotal, research, multiple opinions and single author opinion.
2. Access one of the three models above Crombie (1996), Cormack (2006) and Cottrell (2005) and use it to critically evaluate a piece of research that relates to your area of study.

Stage five: integrating literature

This stage concerns the integration of literature in order to make your arguments stronger. One piece of evidence may have many strengths and may add great support to your position but, for every piece of evidence that supports your stance, there will be many that do not. The critical writer objectively compares and contrasts the variety of works available. It is assumed that if one can critically evaluate one study one can critically evaluate several together; however, integrating literature is a very skilful task that gets easier with practice.

In this stage, the student should identify commonalities and differences in each piece of work and try to explain why they agree and why they differ. The student should also look for any gaps and try to explain them. In this way, the student is looking for order in the chaos. It is easy for students to commit two major sins in this stage, which may be viewed in terms of 'sunny day syndrome' and 'focus on the rain and forget the rainbow'. In the first one the student selects only those pieces of evidence that support their viewpoint and ignores those that don't. This results in students giving a biased view and limits the extent to which they can form arguments. In the second one students select all of the evidence but try to discredit those pieces that disagree with their viewpoint by highlighting all of their weaknesses and ignoring any strengths. This results in partial and flawed arguments. Most markers can easily identify these sins in an essay and this is usually reflected in the grade given.

Stage six: reflection

In this stage, the student should reflect on all of the given information and draw informed conclusions about the soundness of the arguments. Basically, the student pulls all of the information together in order to form some new thinking or theory. The new thinking may support their original idea or may cause the student to have a completely new point of view. Reflection has a second dimension that involves the student reflecting upon the soundness of not only what they have read but also what they have written in their own assignments. A useful framework for evaluating essays can be found in Cottrell (2005) on page 196.

CONCLUSION

This chapter has discussed the importance of critical thinking for students. The first section identified the rationales for critical thinking and stressed that critical thinking is not just about getting better marks but is a lifelong transferable skill. Success in every aspect of human life is tied to the ability to think critically. It is important to acknowledge this, as learning does not end at the end of a course. The second section examined the nature of critical thinking and claimed that it is about moving away from description in order to be more open-minded and questioning. A six-stage model was then proposed that students can use as a framework to direct their approach to critical thinking.

Finally, critical thinking is never final and should result in further evaluation as new knowledge becomes known. Southon and Braithwaite (1998) claim that the ability to think critically in the midst of action and uncertainty is the hallmark of skilled performance and professional behaviour.

Summary

- To critically evaluate health and social care practice, students must develop critical thinking skills.

- Critical analysis is not the same as criticism, the former creates learning and the latter stops it.

- A systematic approach to reviewing the available literature can be found in the six-stage approach.

11

CVs and Interview Techniques

Angela Hastings, Jessica Henderson and
Andrea Hilditch

Learning outcomes

In this chapter you will learn how to:

- complete an application form;

- prepare for a job interview;

- complete a Curriculum Vitae (CV) and covering letter.

INTRODUCTION

It is inevitable that you will at some point need to go for a job interview. For example, you may be applying for your first job following qualification and thereafter applying for different jobs throughout your career. An interview is a way of checking if you are the right person for the job and to establish whether you are a skilled and capable practitioner (Banks, 2002). Going for a job interview is a stressful experience. Nevertheless, you can learn and acknowledge that for each interview experience preparation is important. Sometimes though, you can devote a lot of time to preparation and not be successful, or do very little and hit the jackpot. Interviewing is not an exact science and there are various factors that influence the final outcome – some of these factors are in your control and others are out of your hands. There are, however, some aspects you can prepare for. This chapter will look at ways in which you can prepare yourself for a job interview. Firstly you need to build your self-confidence for the interview day, believe in yourself and understand the whole process of the interviewing game.

WHERE TO BEGIN?

You have seen a job advert online, for example at **www.jobs.nhs.uk** (accessed 11 June 2008) or **www.communitycare.co.uk** (accessed 11 June 2008) and you have decided you want to apply for the job. Usually, within a job advert there will be an identified named person you can contact for an informal discussion about the advertised job (this could be the department manager). The contact person is there to give informal advice and information about the job. Use this person as a first point of call to give you more details. This is a valuable tip: by contacting the named person you may be able to arrange a short visit to the workplace area so that you can find out more and observe the team in action. You will normally be able to meet some of the staff and see for yourself how the team functions, so you may get a 'gut' reaction about the workplace area. If you cannot make a contact visit prior to interview do not worry, but still make the contact with the named person for an informal chat. This contact may give you an idea about the main issues and day-to-day responsibilities of the workplace area. Talking to the named person may be the ideal contact but there are other ways of finding out about the job you have applied for. If this is your first job, ask the other staff too prior to interview. Part of the interviewing process is the fact that you have to go through a decision-making process too – i.e., a key part of this process is deciding whether this is the right job for you. Remember that interviewing is a two-way process; you interview the department just as they interview you. Even if they offer you the post, you still have the option to choose if you will accept it or not.

Completing the application form

Once you have made enquiries about the employer and have been on an informal visit to the work area you will be more aware of the day-to-day responsibilities involved. You are now ready to complete the application form. Many National Health Service (NHS) Trusts in England and Wales now provide online application forms at **www.jobs.nhs.uk**. Take some time to look at this useful website. Social work jobs are advertised in the *Community Care* journal and can be found at **www.communitycare.co.uk/ jobs** (accessed 11 June 2008). For some jobs you will need to apply for the job directly via the Human Resources (HR) Department and the application form is usually sent to you. If you are on a short deadline, you could arrange to pick up the application form from the HR Department.

> ### Activity
>
> Whether completing a written or online application, you will need to consider the following points.
>
> - Ensure you are really interested in the advertised job.
> - Make sure it is an area of work you want to focus upon.
> - Read the job description and person specification – and then consider:
>   (a) if you have the necessary qualities to apply for the job;
>   (b) if you have the qualifications to apply for the job.

If, after all these considerations, you still feel you are a suitable candidate then continue with the process. There appears to be a lot of work to do but if you put the effort in you can become an outstanding candidate.

Online and written applications

For the online and written application the following information should be included in your 'interview pack':

- job reference number;
- job title;
- area of work;
- employer;
- department;
- location;
- salary;
- working pattern – for example, 30 hours;
- job type – for example, temporary or permanent;
- pay scheme;
- closing date – for example, 10th February 2009.

Additional information:

- named contact person;
- job description;
- additional information;
- applicant guidance notes (online);
- information about completing a Criminal Records Bureau (CRB) form;

- information about work permits;
- information about the need to have UK professional registration.

Remember to read all the information.

PREPARING FOR THE JOB INTERVIEW

We begin with the following activity.

Activity

What made you decide you wanted to work in your chosen profession? List your ideas. Keep this list and incorporate your ideas into your application form.

You have made enquiries with the named person, organised a visit to the workplace area and you still want to apply for the job. This is when you apply online or directly with the identified HR Department. A person specification form usually accompanies the application form. You will need to match your skills and experience to the person specification requirements. If you are able to do this the next stage of the process is the completion of the application form and/or the submission of a Curriculum Vitae (CV). Read the advert and write what is asked of you. This can seem like a tedious task but is a very important part of the whole process. The decision to move you to the next stage of the interviewing process depends on the quality of your completed application form or your CV. These will be 'assessed' by the short-listing panel and they will select the best candidates for the interview based on the quality of your application form or your CV. Your application form needs to be an excellent attempt at selling yourself – you are competing against other candidates and therefore need to shine.

Activity

Jane was preparing for her first job interview. She had been asked to deliver a short presentation as part of the interview. What tips would you give Jane to help her prepare for this job interview? (More information on presentation skills can be found in Chapter 7.)

You have thought about the main preparation required for the interview and made a few notes. Did your ideas match the following suggestions?

Remember not to focus on the presentation only. Jane will need to give an 'all round' interview performance. Going for an interview can be compared to undertaking a short oral examination so she needs to prepare; this means anticipating what might be asked at the interview. After visiting the workplace area, talking to other staff, gathering relevant information and reading the job description, Jane may have some idea about what to focus her preparation on. It may be useful to think of any topical issues or recent Government reports that may be relevant to the work area.

Your application form will be scrutinised so be careful if it is handwritten. Your writing must be legible and you should have no alterations. If you word process your application form or complete the online application form, take care to proofread the form and correct any spelling mistakes before you submit it. The presentation of your work needs to be of a high standard. If you submit a poorly presented application form you may not be short-listed. The first sift of applicants is usually based on the quality and content of the application form. You need to catch the eye of the prospective employer (Sharples, 2007).

The section about yourself and why you want to apply for the job is your chance to show off. Never give a negative answer about your skills, capabilities or personality. As part of your preparation for the job, you could do a SWOT analysis (Strengths, Weaknesses, Opportunities and Threats) about yourself prior to the interview but, obviously, you want to focus on your strengths (see also Chapter 9, page 128).

Activity

Have a go at doing your own SWOT analysis. Remember to include the positive comments you have received from placements and in your personal family life.

This can be difficult as we naturally tend to focus on negative attributes rather than positive ones. For example, your strengths may include good communication skills and being good at working as part of a team. Some of your personal attributes may be transferable into the post you are applying for. One example of a transferable skill is that you positively manage your financial situation. Many people juggle paying the bills and work extra hours to pay the rent or mortgage, etc. This attribute would transfer into a new appointment, as many employers ask for someone who is conscious about managing the work area budget. You need to market yourself as the best person for the job. Therefore, take time before the interview to prepare and think about your personal strengths. Consider that you can always turn negative issues into positive issues but this needs practice. You need to be mindful about the possibility of being asked about your personal strengths or weaknesses.

Example

Making a weakness sound like a positive attribute

Interviewer: 'Can you give an example of a personal weakness?'
Candidate: 'I really am aware that I can be overenthusiastic and always want to be involved with all sorts of tasks. This means I get everything done but sometimes I end up doing everyone else's work. I have started to recognise this and am trying to address this by concentrating on my own work tasks.'

Possible interview questions

The actual job interview involves asking you questions, so one way you can attempt to prepare is by thinking about the types of question the interview panel may ask you. Make sure you are familiar with the latest topical issues by reading the relevant press, research and journals (Phillips, 2007). You may be asked to relate these issues to placement areas. The next box includes examples of other possible types of question you may be asked.

Example

Frequently asked questions

- Tell us a little bit about yourself as a person.
- What aspect of your course have you enjoyed most and why?
- Can you tell us about a piece of research that you have found really interesting and learned from?
- How do you ensure effective communication takes place in the care setting?
- Where do you see yourself in five years' time?
- What qualities do you have to bring to this job?
- Why are you the best candidate for the job?
- You may be asked a question about a work situation and how you would deal with it, for example, risk management, a safety issue, a drug error, conflict at work.

It may be difficult as a newly qualified professional to be able to evaluate the experience you have gained. However, you need to think about the placement areas where you have worked during your course and reflect on the main responsibilities of the qualified staff in each area. As a newly qualified professional you will need to consider your future career pathway and think about why you have chosen to apply for this particular job.

Deciding on your first job – where to choose . . . and why?

You need to be conscious that your first job may shape your future career. Choose well and this will help you to consolidate all the learning that has taken place during your training. However, in some instances you may not have the luxury of choice as vacancies can be few and far between. You therefore need to think about how each job advertised will help you develop. If you have worked in a particular placement area you will already have some 'inside information' on some departments or you may be drawn to a particular speciality and therefore be prepared to move locations in order to work in a specialist field. These factors are all part of the interview process. You have to consider all variables as this is a huge decision.

Activity

Decision-making criteria – why do you want this job?

- Think of why you like certain work areas.
- What do you have to offer?
- How can you develop?
- How will this job help your career pathway?

Knowing why you want to work in a particular work area will help to focus your mind. Being unsure as to why you are applying for a job can potentially be reflected at interview (if you get through the short-listing process).

Practise makes perfect

If you have the opportunity to attend a 'mock' interview then do take it. In a mock interview situation you would normally apply for an imaginary job so that you have a chance to practise completing an application form, understanding and reading a job description and presenting yourself in an imaginary interview situation. This will mean you will have to dress appropriately and be conscious of your body language. This is an excellent chance to think about how you present yourself. Attending interviews is stressful and it is normal to be nervous. It is good to experience these feelings, to practise answering questions and, more importantly, to learn how to sell yourself. Receiving feedback on your good and bad points will be helpful to you in the long run.

Tips to help you get through the interview

Influence the situation by presenting yourself well as the interview panel will be influenced by first impressions.

> **Example**
>
> **First impressions – the impact you make**
>
> - You will need to be dressed smartly.
> - Make sure your hair is tidy.
> - Smile, try not to look frightened.
> - Make eye contact with the interview panel.
> - You may want to shake hands with members of the interview panel.
> - When seated be aware of your body language and sit in an 'open' posture – for example, keep your hands on your lap.
> - Listen to the questions and answer articulately.
> - Keep calm.

Act in a relaxed manner and compose yourself. The interview panel is not trying to catch you out; they are looking for the right person for the job. Normally the first couple of questions will be about yourself to help you relax. However, you need to be conscious of what you say and be prepared to expand on any answer you give or in relation to what you have written on your application form.

Getting the most out of yourself

Remember to practise and be prepared for the interview. This includes factors such as knowing what you are going to wear in advance of the interview day and knowing where the interview will take place. If your interview does involve you doing a presentation then you need to practise beforehand – for example, time your presentation, use visual aids as they make the presentation more interesting, ensure you are aware of your eye-to-eye contact with interview panel members (Redfern Jones, 2006) (see also Chapter 7 on Presentations). On the interview day be conscious of your body language including, for example, your posture. You need to portray a calm and confident manner through positive body language and an open posture will portray this. Meet the interview panel with a smile. This always gives you a positive aura. During the interview, speak clearly and slowly so the panel can hear and absorb your answers.

Communicating with the panel by answering the question asked is a key part of the interview process. If you are unsure about a question you have been asked just take your time, rather than replying, 'I can't answer that' or 'I don't know.' Compose yourself by asking the member of the panel to repeat or rephrase the question and, while this is happening, you can be composing your answer. Take deep breaths, apply your personal relaxation technique and keep a positive outlook. Try not to let nerves get the better of you.

Prior to the interview, you can also prepare the questions you want to ask the panel at the end of the interview. It is a good idea to ask about the induction programme the workplace area can offer you, or about professional development opportunities. Preparation in all aspects will help build your confidence.

Example

Body language – don'ts:

- don't fidget with your hair or jewellery;
- don't cross your arms or sit with your handbag on your lap;
- don't sit on the edge of the chair and rock.

Answering questions – don'ts:

- when you are being asked a question don't interrupt the interviewer;
- don't say 'I can't answer that' or 'I don't know';
- don't give one-word answers, unless the question specifically requires a one-word answer.

A GUIDE TO CURRICULUM VITAE (CV) WRITING AND COVERING LETTERS

So, the time has come when you need to prepare a CV. You may have a lot of questions running through your mind: 'What makes a great CV?', 'Where do I start?', 'What do I do about a covering letter?' Hopefully, the following guide should be a useful starting point. Read it first and then try to put together a draft of your CV.

The basics – what is a CV and what is it for?

The literal translation of a Curriculum Vitae (CV) is:

noun (*pl.* curricula vitae) a brief account of a person's education, qualifications, and previous occupations, sent with a job application. – ORIGIN Latin, 'course of (one's) life'.

Merriam Webster Online Dictionary (2008)

Sounds fairly straightforward? There is actually a bit more to a CV than this. It does need careful thought and planning, and is certainly worth taking the time and effort to do properly. A CV is essentially a selling tool as it is the first impression a potential employer will have of you. It should be quick and interesting to read as it is your chance to persuade them to interview you – so make it count! First of all, of course, you need to find out if a CV is required for the job you are applying for.

Example

When should I use a CV?

A CV should be used when:

- specifically asked for in an advertisement;
- the advertisement says 'apply in writing';
- making speculative applications;
- no other method of application has been specified;
- when attending Recruitment and Careers fairs.

A CV should not be used when:

- the advertisement states that CVs will not be accepted.

If in doubt contact the person advertising the job.

What makes a good CV?

A good CV should be:

- **Targeted** – you need to research thoroughly each job you apply for and target your CV so that it is relevant and presents you in the best possible way for each different job.

- **Accurate** – there is no excuse for having poor spelling or grammar.
- **Easy to read** – use clear headings, bullet points, and space your text well but don't overuse layout features and don't use text boxes or tables.
- **Informative but concise** – potential employers don't want to read pages and pages of information.

What should a CV include?

There is a certain amount of flexibility about what sections you should include in your CV. Having said this, some sections are essential and others are optional. Here are some suggestions you may want to consider – these are marked:

(E) = Essential
(O) = Optional

One of the first things to point out is that you don't need to write 'Curriculum Vitae' or 'CV' as a title – it's obvious that it is a CV and writing this just takes up vital space.

Personal details (E)

- **Name (E)** – this should be at the very top – make sure it stands out from the rest of the text. You don't need to repeat this anywhere else.
- **Contact details (E)** – make it as easy as possible for a potential employer to contact you. Include your address, telephone and/or mobile number and e.mail address. If you provide an e.mail address, make sure it is a 'sensible' one – 'sexysusan@msn.com' just isn't professional.
- **Other personal details (O)** – the following details are optional, as it is now illegal to discriminate on this basis – date of birth, nationality and gender. However, there may be some exceptions for specific jobs where it would be acceptable to request this information.

Career objective/personal profile (O)

This is an optional section, but can be a useful way to grab the potential employer's attention. If you use it, keep it brief (no longer than a couple of sentences) and use it as a way to highlight your relevant key skills – don't just include it for the sake of it.

Education (E)

Use reverse chronological order (i.e. most recent first). Only include education from age 16 onwards and include:

- dates – start and finish year;
- university name and location;
- degree course name – you may also include a few relevant modules, projects or your dissertation title. If your dissertation or final year project is relevant to the post applied for, you may want to expand on this. Also include degree results – actual or expected;
- college/school name(s) and location(s);
- for earlier qualifications, you can summarise results together to save space, for example, '8 GCSEs Grades B–C, including English and Maths' (or equivalent qualifications if you studied abroad) and 'A Levels Art (A), English (B), French (B)'.

Employment and work experience and/or career history (E)

Some people worry that they have little or no 'work experience'. Remember that undertaking voluntary work or involvement in groups, societies and/or other activities can also provide great examples of your skills and experience. The purpose of this section is to highlight your relevant experience and skills developed, paying particular attention to any specific responsibilities or achievements:

- 'employment, work experience or career history' – you could use any of these titles for this section – again, use reverse chronological order;
- dates – start and finish month and year and, if the employment was short-term, specify why – for example, a temporary, fixed-term or short-term contract;
- employer name and location – full address is not needed;
- job title;
- responsibilities – either use bullet points, or a short, punchy paragraph – a potential employer will be interested in your individual skills and experiences so think of particular achievements and skills you have developed and the ways in which these are relevant to the vacancy in question;
- you may wish to use separate headings for 'relevant' and 'other' experience, particularly if you have a considerable employment history, as this enables you to provide details on your relevant job(s) and summarise other employment in a shorter section.

Skills and additional information (O)

This can be a useful way to include any other information not covered elsewhere. For example, driving-licence, IT skills (such as packages used, level of competence), languages and any other skills or qualifications.

Interests (O)

This is a way to demonstrate your personality and individuality and yet another way to evidence skills.

Referees (E)

Always obtain permission from the individual before nominating them as a referee. Keep them updated about any jobs you may be applying for.

Layout

- Normally, a CV should be no more than two pages but exceptions can be made for academic CVs and performers.
- Keep it clear and simple – avoid fancy fonts and graphics – look at the way we have laid out this chapter for ways of formatting your CV.
- Make sure you don't split important points over two pages.
- Put your most relevant selling points on the first page for the most impact.

Example

Practical checklist – the DOs:
- Have you remembered to accompany your CV with a covering letter?
- Is your CV clear, easy to read and spell-checked? Ask a friend to look at it for you.
- Check the alignment of paragraphs.
- Ask yourself, 'Would my CV and covering letter make an impact on me if I were the employer?' and 'Is my CV tailored to the job description?'

And the DON'Ts:
- Don't staple pages together.
- Don't forget, if you are posting your CV, use the correct amount of postage. You don't want to go to all that effort only for your CV to be delayed in the post or not reach the employer just because you have not used the correct postage.

The covering letter

So, you now have a first-class CV and are ready to send off your application. How do you ensure that:

- it gets to the right person and
- they take the time to read it?

This is where your covering letter comes in. A good covering letter should be brief – usually no more than one side of A4 – but provide enough information to impress the employer and encourage them to find out more about you by reading your CV or application form. It should:

- **introduce you** – tell them why you are writing, where you saw the opportunity advertised and, if you are making a speculative application, the type of work you are seeking;

- **show that you have done your research** – i.e., the letter should demonstrate why you are interested in this type of work and that you have an understanding of what it is likely to involve;

- **be targeted** – i.e., the letter should explain why you are interested in working for this particular organisation so you need to find out as much about them as you can and demonstrate an understanding of their sector of work;

- **sell you** – the letter should explain what makes you better than other applicants, but don't repeat what is in your CV or application form; use this as an opportunity to draw the employer's attention to a few key skills and experiences that make you the ideal candidate for the role.

- **deal with problem areas** – take the opportunity, if necessary, to explain any anomalies in your CV, such as gaps, or any areas where you do not match the selection criteria, but remember to explain any anomalies in the most positive way possible, for example, give details of how you overcame any hurdles;

- **end positively** – indicate your availability for interview and end the letter on a positive note – for example, 'I look forward to discussing my application with you in more detail.'

Example

Covering letter – do:

- address it to the right person;
- use professional language and layout;
- end it correctly – if you address the letter to a named person, such as 'Mr Jones', you should end it 'Yours sincerely'. If the letter is addressed to 'Sir/Madam' end it 'Yours faithfully';
- word process it (unless the advert specifically states otherwise).

Don't:

- Fall into the e.mail trap – an electronic covering letter should be as professional as a 'hard' copy letter.

When should you use a covering letter?

- Always when sending a CV.
- Optionally with application forms.
- When making speculative applications.
- When asked to make a 'letter of application'.

CONCLUSION

Remember that your CV needs to be kept up to date. It can be adapted to whatever job you are applying for and there is no definitive way of structuring it. The format chosen depends on the information you want to impart.

This chapter has explored the topics of how to complete an application form, prepare for a job interview, put together your curriculum vitae (CV) and write your covering letter. Please note, this chapter is provided as a study aid and these are suggestions only. It is in no way a guarantee that you will obtain work if you follow the information provided. However, use the chapter as an *aide-mémoire* to help you towards your goal of achieving employment.

Summary

- A carefully prepared application form will help you get to the interview stage.

- Good preparation and body language will give the right impression at interview.

- Your CV should include all the information that will sell your skills.

- A covering letter provides a brief synopsis of why you should be considered suitable for the job.

Appendix

QAA (2001) Qualification descriptors

Descriptor for a qualification at Certificate (C) level: Certificate of Higher Education

Certificates of Higher Education are awarded to students who have demonstrated:

i) knowledge of the underlying concepts and principles associated with their area(s) of study, and an ability to evaluate and interpret these within the context of that area of study;

ii) an ability to present, evaluate, and interpret qualitative and quantitative data, to develop lines of argument and make sound judgements in accordance with basic theories and concepts of their subject(s) of study.

Typically, holders of the qualification will be able to:

a) evaluate the appropriateness of different approaches to solving problems related to their area(s) of study and/or work;

b) communicate the results of their study/work accurately and reliably, and with structured and coherent arguments;

c) undertake further training and develop new skills within a structured and managed environment;

and will have:

d) qualities and transferable skills necessary for employment requiring the exercise of some personal responsibility.

Descriptor for a qualification at Intermediate (I) level: Degree (non-Honours)

Non-Honours degrees are awarded to students who have demonstrated:

i) knowledge and critical understanding of the well-established principles of their area(s) of study, and of the way in which those principles have developed;

ii) ability to apply underlying concepts and principles outside the context in which they were first studied, including, where appropriate, the application of those principles in an employment context;

iii) knowledge of the main methods of enquiry in their subject(s), and ability to evaluate critically the appropriateness of different approaches to solving problems in the field of study;

iv) an understanding of the limits of their knowledge, and how this influences analyses and interpretations based on that knowledge.

Typically, holders of the qualification will be able to:

a) use a range of established techniques to initiate and undertake critical analysis of information, and to propose solutions to problems arising from that analysis;

b) effectively communicate information, arguments and analysis, in a variety of forms, to specialist and non-specialist audiences, and deploy key techniques of the discipline effectively;

c) undertake further training, develop existing skills, and acquire new competences that will enable them to assume significant responsibility within organisations;

and will have:

d) qualities and transferable skills necessary for employment requiring the exercise of personal responsibility and decision-making.

Descriptor for a qualification at Honours (H) level: Bachelor's degree with Honours

Honours degrees are awarded to students who have demonstrated:

i) a systematic understanding of key aspects of their field of study, including acquisition of coherent and detailed knowledge, at least some of which is at, or informed by, the forefront of defined aspects of a discipline;

ii) an ability to deploy accurately established techniques of analysis and enquiry within a discipline;

iii) conceptual understanding that enables the student:
- to devise and sustain arguments, and/or to solve problems, using ideas and techniques, some of which are at the forefront of a discipline; and
- to describe and comment upon particular aspects of current research, or equivalent advanced scholarship, in the discipline;

iv) an appreciation of the uncertainty, ambiguity and limits of knowledge;

v) the ability to manage their own learning, and to make use of scholarly reviews and primary sources (e.g. refereed research articles and/or original materials appropriate to the discipline).

Typically, holders of the qualification will be able to:
a) apply the methods and techniques that they have learned to review, consolidate, extend and apply their knowledge and understanding, and to initiate and carry out projects;
b) critically evaluate arguments, assumptions, abstract concepts and data (that may be incomplete), to make judgements, and to frame appropriate questions to achieve a solution – or identify a range of solutions – to a problem;
c) communicate information, ideas, problems, and solutions to both specialist and non-specialist audiences;

and will have:
d) qualities and transferable skills necessary for employment requiring:
   - the exercise of initiative and personal responsibility;
   - decision-making in complex and unpredictable contexts; and
   - the learning ability needed to undertake appropriate further training of a professional or equivalent nature.

Descriptor for a qualification at Master's (M) level: Master's degree

Master's degrees are awarded to students who have demonstrated:
i) a systematic understanding of knowledge, and a critical awareness of current problems and/or new insights, much of which is at, or informed by, the forefront of their academic discipline, field of study, or area of professional practice;
ii) a comprehensive understanding of techniques applicable to their own research or advanced scholarship;
iii) originality in the application of knowledge, together with a practical understanding of how established techniques of research and enquiry are used to create and interpret knowledge in the discipline;
iv) conceptual understanding that enables the student:
   - to evaluate critically current research and advanced scholarship in the discipline; and
   - to evaluate methodologies and develop critiques of them and, where appropriate, to propose new hypotheses.

Typically, holders of the qualification will be able to:
a) deal with complex issues both systematically and creatively, make sound judgements in the absence of complete data, and communicate their conclusions clearly to specialist and non-specialist audiences;
b) demonstrate self-direction and originality in tackling and solving

problems, and act autonomously in planning and implementing tasks at a professional or equivalent level;

c) continue to advance their knowledge and understanding, and to develop new skills to a high level;

and will have:

d) the qualities and transferable skills necessary for employment requiring:
   - the exercise of initiative and personal responsibility;
   - decision-making in complex and unpredictable situations; and
   - the independent learning ability required for continuing professional development.

Descriptor for qualifications at Doctoral (D) level: Doctoral degree

Doctorates are awarded to students who have demonstrated:

i) the creation and interpretation of new knowledge, through original research or other advanced scholarship, of a quality to satisfy peer review, extend the forefront of the discipline, and merit publication;

ii) a systematic acquisition and understanding of a substantial body of knowledge which is at the forefront of an academic discipline or area of professional practice;

iii) the general ability to conceptualise, design and implement a project for the generation of new knowledge, applications or understanding at the forefront of the discipline, and to adjust the project design in the light of unforeseen problems;

iv) a detailed understanding of applicable techniques for research and advanced academic enquiry.

Typically, holders of the qualification will be able to:

a) make informed judgements on complex issues in specialist fields, often in the absence of complete data, and be able to communicate their ideas and conclusions clearly and effectively to specialist and non-specialist audiences;

b) continue to undertake pure and/or applied research and development at an advanced level, contributing substantially to the development of new techniques, ideas, or approaches;

and will have:

c) the qualities and transferable skills necessary for employment requiring the exercise of personal responsibility and largely autonomous initiative in complex and unpredictable situations, in professional or equivalent environments.

The Quality Assurance Agency (2006) Subject benchmark statements for health and social care

1 Values in health and social care practice

Health and social care professionals are personally accountable for their actions and must be able to explain and justify their decisions. They work in many different settings and practices and have to make difficult decisions about complex human situations, which require the application of ethical principles. They seek to improve the quality of life for their patients and clients. All hold a duty to protect and promote the needs of their clients and patients and, in so doing, take into account any associated risks for the public.

1.1 Respect for clients' and patients' rights, individuality, dignity and privacy

Health and social care staff should:

- be open and honest with their clients and patients;
- listen to clients and patients;
- keep information about clients and patients confidential within the limits of duty of care;
- ensure that their own beliefs do not prejudice the care of their clients and patients;
- recognise and value cultural and social diversity;
- ensure individualised care and treatment to combat discrimination and social exclusion.

1.2 Clients' and patients' right to be involved in decisions about their health and social care

Health and social care staff should:

- provide information about clients' and patients' health and social care options in a manner in which the clients and patients can understand;
- gain appropriate consent before giving care and treatment;
- enable clients and patients to make informed choices about care, including cases where those choices may result in adverse outcomes for the individual;
- provide clients and patients with proper access to their health and social care records.

1.3 Justify public trust and confidence

Health and social care staff should:

- be honest and trustworthy at all times;
- act with integrity and never abuse their professional standing;
- never ask for or accept any inducement, gift, hospitality or referral which may affect, or be considered to affect, their professional judgement;
- always declare any personal interests to those who may be affected.

1.4 High standards of practice

Health and social care staff should:

- recognise and work within the limits of their knowledge, skills and experience;
- maintain and improve their professional knowledge, skills and performance;
- be committed to enhancing standards of practice in health and social care;
- make prompt, relevant, clear, legible and proper records;
- must deliver the highest standards of integrity and competence.

1.5 Protection from risk of harm

Health and social care staff should:

- act properly to protect clients, patients, the public and colleagues from the risk of harm;
- ensure that their own or their colleagues' health, conduct or performance does not place clients and patients at risk;
- protect clients and patients from risks of infection or other dangers in the environment.

1.6 Co-operation and collaboration with colleagues

Health and social care staff should:

- respect and encourage the skills and contributions which colleagues in both their own profession and other professions bring to the care of clients and patients;
- within their work environment, support colleagues to develop their professional knowledge, skills and performance;
- not require colleagues to take on responsibilities that are beyond their level of knowledge, skills and experience.

1.7 Education

Health and social care staff should, where appropriate:

- contribute to the education of students, colleagues, clients and patients, and the wider public;
- develop skills of responsible and proper supervision.

2 The practice of health and social care

Health and social care are applied academic subjects, where practice is underpinned by theoretical learning. In their practice, health and social care professionals draw from the values, knowledge and skills of their own discipline. This knowledge and understanding forms the basis for making decisions and judgements in a variety of contexts, often against a backdrop of uncertainty. Partnership working is essential to promote the well-being of individuals, groups and communities. Professional practice is essentially a process of problem solving. It can be characterised by four major phases:

- the identification and assessment of health and social care needs in the context of individuals' interaction with their environment;
- the development of focused intervention to meet these needs;
- implementation of these plans;
- critical evaluation of the impact of professional and service interventions on patients and clients.

2.1 Identification and assessment of health and social care needs

Health and social care staff should be able to:

- obtain relevant information from a wide range of sources, using a variety of appropriate assessment methods;
- adopt systematic approaches to evaluating information collected;
- communicate their evaluations effectively to their clients, patients and other members of the health and social care team.

2.2 The development of plans to meet health and social care needs

Health and social care staff should be able to use knowledge, understanding and experience to:

- work with clients and patients to consider the range of activities that are appropriate;
- plan care, and do so holistically;
- record judgements and decisions clearly.

2.3 Implementation of health and social care plans

Health and social care staff should be able to:

- conduct appropriate activities skillfully and in accordance with good practice;
- assign priorities to the work to be done effectively;
- maintain accurate records;
- use opportunities provided by practice to educate others.

2.4 Evaluation of the health and social care plans implemented

Health and social care staff should be able to:

- assess and document the outcomes of their practice;
- involve clients and patients in assessing the effectiveness of the care given;
- learn from their practice to improve the care given in the particular case;
- learn from the experience to improve their future practice;
- participate in audit and other quality assurance procedures to contribute to effective risk management and good clinical governance;
- use the outcomes of evaluation to develop health and social care policy and practice.

2.5 Communication

Health and social care staff should be able to:

- make active, effective and purposeful contact with individuals and organisations utilising appropriate means such as verbal, paper-based and electronic communication;
- build and sustain relationships with individuals, groups and organisations;
- work with others to effect positive change and deliver professional and service accountability.

3 Knowledge and understanding for health and social care practice

The education and training of health and social care professionals draws from a range of academic disciplines which provide the underpinning knowledge and understanding for sound practice. Each profession has an identifiable body of knowledge and will draw from this as appropriate. However, there are areas of knowledge and understanding that are common to all health and social care professionals, which include;

- ethical principles, values and moral concepts inherent in health and social care practice;
- legislation and professional and statutory codes of conduct relevant to their practice, and understanding of health and social care delivery configurations;
- research and evidence-based concepts and explanations from law, psychology, social policy and sociology;
- physical and psychological human growth and development.

In addition, and to an extent determined by the nature of their practice, health and social care professionals will be familiar with:

- the structure, function and dysfunction of the human body;
- public health principles;
- health education in their practice.

References

Alpay, E. (2005) 'Group dynamic processes in e.mail groups'. *Active Learning in Higher Education*, 6 (1): 7–16

Atkins, S. and Murphy, K. (1992) 'Reflection: a review of the literature'. *Journal of Advanced Nursing*, 18: 1188–92

Banks, C. (2002) 'Prepare to succeed'. *Nursing Standard*, 17(5): 96

Beecroft, C., Rees, A., Booth, A. (2006) 'Finding the evidence', in Gerrish K. and Lacey, A. (eds) *The Research Process in Nursing* (5th Ed). Oxford: Blackwell, 90–106

Belbin, M. (1981) *Management Teams: Why they succeed or fail*. London: Butterworth Heinemann

Bell, J. (2006) *Doing your Research Project. A guide for first-time researchers in education, health and social science* (4th Ed). Maidenhead: Open University Press

Benner, P.E. (2001) *From Novice to Expert: excellence and power in nursing practice*. New Jersey: Prentice Hall

Blakeman, K. (2007) *Tricks and tips for better web search* **www.rba.co.uk/wordpress/2007/12/06/presentation-tricks-and-tips-for-better-web-search/** (accessed 16 January 2008)

Blaxter, L., Hughes, C. and Tight, M. (2006) *How to Research* (3rd Ed). Maidenhead: Open University Press

Bradbury, A. (2000) *Successful Presentation Skills* (3rd Ed). London: Kogan Page

Brown, R.A. (1992) *Portfolio Development and Profiling for Nurses*. Lancaster: Quay Publishing Ltd

Burnard, P. (2004) *Writing Skills in Health Care*. Cheltenham: Nelson Thornes

Canter, D. and Fairbairn, G. (2006) *Becoming an Author*. Buckinghamshire: Open University Press

Care Council for Wales (2005) *Standards on Involving Service Users and Carers in Social Work Education*. Cardiff: Welsh Assembly Government

Carper, B. (1978) 'Fundamental patterns of knowing in nursing'. *Advances in Nursing Science*, 1(1): 13–23

Carroll, R. T. (2004) *Becoming a Critical Thinker*. Cambridge: Pearson Custom Publishing

Carvin, A. (2004) 'A quick and easy guide to creative commons licenses'. Digital

Divide Network. **www.digitaldivide.net/articles/view.php?ArticleID=70** (accessed 20 June 2008)

Childs, S. (2003) *Judge: Web sites for health*. Contact a Family and the Information Society Research and Consultancy Group, School of Computing, Engineering and Information Sciences, Northumbria University **www.judgehealth.org.uk** (accessed 20 December 2007)

Coffin, C., Curry, M.J., Goodman, S., Hewings, A., Lillis, T. M. and Swann, J. (2003) *Teaching Academic Writing: A Toolkit for Higher Education*. London: Routledge

Colliver, J. A. (2000) 'Effectiveness of problem based learning curricula: Research and theory'. *Academic Medicine*, 75(3): 259–266

Cormack, D. (2006) *The Research Process in Nursing* (5th Ed). Oxford: Blackwell Publishing

Cottrell, S. (1999) The *Study Skills Handbook*. Basingstoke: Palgrave Macmillan

Cottrell, S. (2001) *The Study Skills Handbook* (2nd Ed). Basingstoke: Palgrave Macmillan

Cottrell, S. (2003) *The Study Skills Handbook* (3rd Ed). Basingstoke: Palgrave Macmillan

Cottrell, S. (2005) *Critical Thinking Skills. Developing effective analysis and argument*. Basingstoke: Palgrave Macmillan

Crombie, I. (1996) *The Pocket Guide to Critical Appraisal: a handbook for health care professionals*. London: British Medical Journal

Crowe, A. (2005) *Speed Reading – Harness your computer's power to triple your reading speed*. Ireland: Cucoco Ltd

Department for Education and Skills (2005) *Common Core of Skills and Knowledge for the Children's Workforce*. Nottingham: DfES Publications

Department of Health (2002) *Requirements for social work training*. London: HMSO

DeYoung, S. (2003) *Teaching Strategies for Nurse Educators*. New Jersey: Prentice Hall

Downs (1993) 'Developing Learning Skills in Vocational Learning', in Thorpe, M., Edwards, E. and Hanson, A. (eds) *Culture and Processes of Adult Learning*. London: Routledge

Drew, S. and Bingham, R. (2001) *The Student Skills Guide*. Aldershot: Gower

Edwards, S. (1998) 'Critical thinking and analysis: A model for written assignments'. *British Journal of Nursing*, 7(3): 159–166

Fry, H., Ketteridge, S. and Marshall, S. (2003) *A Handbook for Teaching and Learning in Higher Education* (2nd Ed). London: Routledge Falmer

General Social Care Council (2002) *Codes of practice for social care workers and codes of practice for employers of social care workers*. London: General Social Care Council

Gibbs, G. (1998) *Learning by Doing: a guide to teaching and learning methods*. Oxford: Oxford Polytechnic

Glen, S. and Leiba, T. (2002) *Multi-professional Learning for Nurses*. Basingstoke: Palgrave

Goleman, D. (1996) *Emotional Intelligence: Why it can matter more than IQ*. London: Bloomsbury

HEFCE (1995) *Report on Quality Assessment* 1992–1995. Higher Education Funding Council for England. Bristol: Northavon House

Honey, P. and Mumford, A. (2006) *Learning Styles Questionnaire*. Maidenhead: Peter Honey Publications

Hull, C., Redfern, L. and Shuttleworth, A. (2005) *Profiles and Portfolios: a guide for health and social care* (2nd Ed). Basingstoke: Palgrave Macmillan

Jasper, M. (2003) *Beginning Reflective Practice: foundations in nursing and health care*. Cheltenham: Nelson Thornes

Johns, C. (2000) *Becoming a Reflective Practitioner: a reflective and holistic approach to clinical nursing, practice development and clinical supervision.* Oxford: Blackwell Science

Knight, P. T. (2007) 'Grading, classifying and future learning'. Chapter 6 in Boud, D. and Falchikof, N. (eds), *Rethinking Assessment in Higher Education: learning for the longer term*. Maidenhead: The Society for Research in Higher Education and the Open University Press

Kolb, D. (1984) *Experiential Learning as the Science of Learning and Development.* New Jersey: Prentice Hall

Lewis, R. (1994) *How to Manage Your Study Time*. Glasgow: Harper Collins

Lindsay, B. (2007) *Understanding Research and Evidence-based Practice*. Exeter: Reflect Press

Linklater, A. (2008) 'My brother's first joint and his descent into a mental war zone'. The *Observer*. Available at **http://observer.guardian.co.uk/society/2008/jan/13/drugsandalcohol.health** (accessed 19 June 2008)

Lloyd, M. (2007) 'Developing academic writing skills: the PROCESS framework'. *Nursing Standard*, 21(40): 50–56

Maslin-Prothero, S. (2002) *Bailliere's Study Skills for Nurses* (2nd Ed). London: Bailliere Tindall

Maslin-Prothero, S. (2005) (ed) *Bailliere's Study Skills for Nurses and Midwives* (3rd Ed). London: Elsevier

Mason-Whitehead, E. and Mason, T. (2008) *Study Skills for Nurses* (2nd Ed). London: Sage Publications

Maznevski, M.L. (1994) 'Undertaking our differences: performance in decision making groups with diverse members?' *Human Relations*, 47(5): 531–552

McCarthy, P. and Hatcher, C. (2002) *Presentation Skills, the Essential Guide for Students.* London: Sage

McClarey, M. and Duff, L. (1997) 'Clinical effectiveness and evidence based practice'. *Nursing Standard*, 11(51): 1–35

Mehrabian, A. (1972) *Nonverbal Communication*. Chicago: Aldine Atherton

Mottola, C. and Murphy, P. (2001) 'Antidote dilemma – an activity to promote critical thinking'. *Journal of Continuing Education in Nursing*, 32(4): 161–164

NAfW (2002) *Fitness for Practice: All Wales Initiative*. Cardiff: National Assembly for Wales

NEWI (2007) *How to do a literature search:* guideline no. 80 **www.newi.ac.uk/en/StudyingatGlyndwr/Studentsupportservices/Libraryandstudy/Guidelines** (accessed 11 June 2008)

NEWI (2007) *Searching the Internet*: guideline no.19. **www.newi.ac.uk/en/**

StudyingatGlyndwr/Studentsupportservices/Libraryandstudy/Guidelines (accessed 14 January 2008)

Nganasurian, W. (1999) *Accreditation of Prior Learning for Nurses and Midwives.* London: Quay Books

Norman, M. and Hyland, T. (2003) 'The role of confidence in lifelong learning'. *Educational Studies*, 29(3). 261–272

Northledge, A. (1994) *The Good Study Guide.* Milton Keynes: Open University Press

O' Dochartaigh, N. (2002) *The Internet Research Handbook: A practical guide for students and researchers in the social sciences.* London: Sage Publications Ltd

Ofcom (2006) The Communications Market Report 2006 **http://www.ofcom.org.uk/research/cm/cm06** (accessed June 2008)

Payne, E. and Whittaker, L. (2000) *Developing Essential Study Skills.* Harlow: Pearson Education

Phillips, S (2007) 'Perfecting your interview technique'. *The Answer*, Spring 2007. London: RCN

Place, E., Kendall, M., Hiom, D., Booth, H., Ayres, P., Manuel, A. and Smith, P. (2006) 'Internet Detective: Wise up to the Web', (3rd Ed), *Intute Virtual Training Suite* [online]. Available from: **www.vts.intute.ac.uk/detective** (accessed 29 August 2007)

Price, B. (2003) *Studying Nursing Using Problem-Based and Enquiry-Based Learning.* London: Palgrave

Proctor, M. (2006) 'Advice on Academic Writing'. University of Toronto. **www.utoronto.ca/writing/advise.html** (accessed 29 August 2007)

Prosser, M. and Trigwell, K. (2001) *Understanding Learning and Teaching.* Buckingham: SRHE and Open University Press

QAA (2001) *The framework for higher education qualifications in England, Wales and Northern Ireland.* **http://www.qaa.ac.uk/academicinfrastructure/fheq/EWNI/default.asp** (accessed June 2008)

QAA (2006a) *Code of Practice for the assurance of standards and quality in higher education, Section 6, assessment of students.* Quality Assurance Agency

QAA (2006b) *Statement of common purpose for subject benchmark statements for the health and social care professions.* **http://www.qaa.ac.uk/academicinfrastructure/benchmark/health/StatementofCommonPurpose06.asp** (accessed June 2008)

QAA (2006c) *Academic credit in higher education in England.* Mansfield: Quality Assurance Agency

Quinn, F. M. (2000) *Principles and Practice of Nurse Education.* London: Nelson Thornes

Ramsden, P. (2005) Editorial. *Academy Exchange*, 2: 3

Redfern Jones, J. (2006) 'Stand and Deliver' *Nursing Standard*, 21(6): 64

Regan, J. (2003) 'Motivating students towards self-directed learning' *Nurse Education Today*, 23: 593–599

Rolfe, G. (2000) *Research, Truth, Authority.* Basingstoke: Palgrave Macmillan

Rose, J. (2001) *The Mature Student's Guide to Writing.* Basingstoke: Palgrave

Schafersman, S. D. (1991) *An introduction to critical thinking.* Available at **www.freeinquiry.com/critical-thinking.html** (accessed 9 January 2008)

Sharples, K. (2007) 'Are you just the job?' *Nursing Standard*, 21(40): 61

Silverman, D. (2006) *Interpreting Qualitative Data* (3rd Ed). London: Sage

Singh, V. (2002) 'Managing Diversity for Strategic Advantage' – Conference Report. London: Council for Excellence in Management and Leadership

Southon, G. and Braithwaite, J. (1998) 'The end of professionalism?' *Social Science and Medicine*, 46(1): 23–28

Stephenson, S. (2000) *Exemplars of reflection*, cited in Bulman, C. and Schutz, S. (eds) (2004) *Reflective Practice in Nursing* (3rd Ed). Oxford: Blackwell

Stone, P.W. (2002) 'Popping the (PICO) question in research and evidence based practice'. *Applied Nursing Research*, 15(3): 197–8

Sullivan, E. and Decker, P. (1997) *Effective Leadership and Management in Nursing* (4th Ed). Menlo Park: Addison-Wesley

Thompson, N. (2000) *Understanding Social Work: Preparing for Practice.* Basingstoke: Palgrave

Thompson, N. (2003) *Communication and Language: a handbook of theory and practice.* Basingstoke: Palgrave

TOPSS (2002) *National Occupational Standards – The key purpose and key roles of social work* **www.topssengland.net/files/cd/England/Main.htm** (accessed 3 March 2008)

Truelove, S. (2003) *Intellectual Thinkers on Training.* Stockport: Institute of Training and Occupational Learning

Tuckman, B.W. (1965) 'Developmental sequences in small groups'. *Psychological Bulletin*, 63: 384–399

UK©CS (2004) Factsheet PO-1: *UK Copyright Law.* The UK Copyright Service. **www.copyrightservice.co.uk/copyright/p01_uk_copyright_law** (accessed 29 August 2007)

van Emden, J. and Becker, L. (2004) *Presentation Skills for Students.* Basingstoke: Palgrave Macmillan

van Gelder, T. (2004) 'Teaching critical thinking. Some lessons from cognitive science'. *College Teaching*, 45: 1–6

Warren (2007) *Service User and Carer Participation in Social Work.* Exeter: Learning Matters

Wilkie, K. and Burns, I. (2003) *Problem-Based Learning: A Handbook for Nurses.* Basingstoke: Palgrave

Websites

Plagiarism – **www.plagiarism.org** (accessed11 June 2008)

Internet Detective – **www.vts.intute.ac.uk/detective** (accessed 2 June 2008)

Merriam Webster Online Dictionary – www.merriam-webster.com (accessed 18 July 2008)

Online Writing Lab – (OWL) **www.owl.english.purdue.edu** (accessed 11 June 2008)

Readpal™ – **www.readpal.com** (accessed 11 June 2008)

Index